SING TO ME
WHILE I CAN HEAR

memoirs of a caregiver

and the evolution of a mother/daughter relationship

JODY LEWIS

for my children
with the hope that they see
that even unto old age
love may thrive in fragile places
where it had not grown before

White Canoe Productions

ISBN 0-9772115-0-9

Printed in the United States by
Independent Publishing Corporation
St. Louis, Missouri 63011

Contents

Contents, continued

Introduction

In January of 1998, my mother awoke and went to the kitchen to begin preparing dinner for ten for that evening. She probably proceeded in her usual efficient way– starting the defrosting of the meat for the entree, planning her shopping list for fresh vegetables, putting the vacuum cleaner where she would be sure not to overlook it as the day went on. She took a break to go bathe; and when she emerged, she started to continue her plan of action. She did not get very far into her program, because with horrifying swiftness her mind went blank. She must have started to say something out loud to herself, but she heard nothing recognizable as either her words or her voice. She had the presence of mind to get to the phone and call her younger daughter, dialing numbers that worked for her for almost the last time; and in a voice of fear and confusion, struggling to say that something was wrong, she repeated over and over again essentially incoherent phrases. They served the purpose and got both her daughter and an ambulance speeding to her. My mother was eighty-seven, just two months short of eighty-eight, in outstanding health until that minute when it would never be true again. She had had a major stroke and dinner for ten would be, forever after, out of her power.

My relationship with my mother had not been sullen or stormy; it had been difficult in other ways. She had wanted a daughter just like her but got someone very different, just as I would have preferred a very different kind of mother. We seemed to fall into a gray area that could not really be called a love/hate relationship, staying much cooler in both directions. It was a sort-of-respect/sort-of-dislike seesaw that we rode. She felt personally rejected; I felt unknown and diminished. Our journey together in this new relationship of her degree of need and my degree of willingness to meet that need went along a very uneven path. This collection of essays and poems is about that journey; but it is offered in a spirit of saying, "If you are in a similar situation, perhaps I can be of help." I hope my words can clarify your own on days when it is too hard even to know what you think. I hope the poems written as if by my mother will offer another angle of understanding in what you are going through, though many people will need no outside voice.

I have given careful thought to the degree of openness I should allow into this memoir of our experiences together. Should I spare the more physical details of caregiving? Should I write as if it were easy? I have opted for sharing the reality, but it is not all grim. For all the frustration and anguish, there are many pleasures. There is fun. I hope you will find it worthwhile to be a guest in an array of our experiences.

Sing To Me ~ ~

Ghost is was.
My bain be fuzz.
I see the nothness in my head.

I feel dark spaces, bleakly places,
behind my eyes. Blank faces
me. I soon be dead.

Sometize I watch the feathers fall
from three tall trees and more of these
than I remezzer how to counts.

I watch the days go ounce by ounce
and sleep away the longly nights.
I miss my love, my young man love;
what was his name? He be my knight,
my king, my was.
Like mine, his bain be fuzz.

Oh, empy, empy in my hood;
profound I do not see.
It all come round invisibly,
ice roses where my brain has bled.
It be no good.

Now sing to me while I can hear,
and I will song you too.
Be night, be night, I go home now.
Tell me if I love you.

Institutional Walls

It would be irresponsible of me to claim that no one belongs in hospitals or nursing homes. There are so many reasons that our current care facilities must exist and must serve a huge range of needs. Still, I have to regard such places with an extremely wary eye and with the adamant conviction that every patient needs a personal advocate in order to receive quality care; and, even then, the odds are not in the patients' favor. Ideally that advocate should be someone personally close to the patient and zealous in his or her behalf.

In this first section, I introduce my mother's initial situation and give a brief picture of what stroke did to her and describe how she was in the four weeks following her stroke. The first week was in two different hospital areas– the neurological wing and then in a general wing. The remaining three weeks were in the sub-acute area where she underwent rehabilitation therapies. Our experience in the first week was constantly frustrating, filled with obstacles, overloaded with miscommunication and disturbing distrust of us from some members of the hospital staff. A large part of the problem was the medical team's interpretation of advocacy as personal criticism of them as individuals and a few mistaken assumptions about our reasons for being present all day long, although it is certainly true that we did want to protect her from some of the harsher personnel. Like professionals in many areas, they tended to regard themselves as the experts on their patients; but it became painfully clear that they were often indifferent to individuals and, therefore, no experts at all. Just as they knew who they were and what they were about without knowing a thing about us or, frankly, about my mother, we knew nothing about them and wanted to learn. Mostly we wanted them to treat her with respect, not as the child she so suddenly had come to appear. One thing is definitely true at this point in history: few people know anything about the way stroke affects the inner lives of its victims. It is neither easy nor wise to trust all strangers, especially when lives are in their hands and they do not even seem aware of that fact. If anyone had ever asked us about the real her instead of merely about the events of the stroke and the symptoms and losses, we might have felt that they were truly wanting to help her. By their constant focus on how she presented herself to them in the current moment, they really could not help her nearly so well.

Details follow. Expect some repetition.

~ Six Hundred Is a Meaningless Number

When I arrived at the hospital about an hour after Mom and my sister did, she was frightened and very aware that something was all wrong, that her mind was not working properly. She still knew that what she was saying was unintelligible, and her frustration was increasing rapidly. Some of her words were recognizable; most were nonsense syllables. Among the recognizable words that were being regarded as essentially meaningless was the recurrent phrase, *six hundred, six hundred, six hundred*. Some of the members of the hospital staff tried to insist that she was saying random sounds, that we should not try to make sense of them, that we should just make soothing sounds to reassure her. We did not all agree with their assessment. The fact that *six hundred* held no specific meaning for them in relation to her hardly meant that it was meaningless. The fortunate fact that I had been helping her keep her financial records for a few years gave me the clue that did make sense of the number and brought her instant relief. She still was in possession of the fact that she had a deadline for a financial transaction that was coming up, and it involved paperwork for an asset that was splitting from three hundred shares to six hundred. For almost a full year after her stroke she would retain a strong hold on the details that mattered to her; and certainly her financial wellbeing was a major component. The moment I asked her if she meant those shares, she relaxed and smiled; and when I assured her that it would be taken care of, she closed her eyes and breathed more easily. The wall we kept running into, though, was the medical staff's insistence that nothing she said could be thought to make sense.

Food and entertaining were also important parts of her life. That first day, once she relaxed from the fear of losing the financial asset, her mind turned to the dinner she had been preparing. Again she struggled to communicate with us, but not one sound that she uttered made any dent in our understanding.

"Pencil," Mom said. The staff smiled patronizingly. Over and over she said that same word. We brought her a pencil; she angrily shoved it aside. "No!" she said quite clearly and adamantly.

"What?" we kept asking.

"Pencil!" she shouted angrily, filled with frustration. We got nowhere. We tried to distract her to another topic: what had she been fixing for dinner? "Pencil!" she declared happily. We tried to move on, but nothing appeased her.

"Is *pencil* dinner?" we joked a little. After all, she had sounded happy.

"Yes!" she insisted. "Get pencil."

"Where is it?" we asked.

"At my pencil!" she said impatiently.

Again the therapists shrugged and insisted we were wasting our energy. There we were, playing a form of "Coffeepot" where all the answers were *pencil*. The nurses and others who came in and out of the room shook their heads. Later several therapists would say more strenuously that we were simply in denial of the truth that Mom had lost her mental faculties. But what did their attitude do for her or for us? Once more, by taking her seriously, we were able to rescue the packages of veal cutlets thawing on her kitchen counter. The moment we connected, however accidentally or jokingly (*is pencil dinner?*) to what she knew she meant, she could relax, could smile, could sleep. We had an advantage that no outside real or self-styled expert possibly can have: we knew her, and we knew that she always did hate waste.

~ Bad Omens

Normally I think that it's a good thing that most of us cannot see into the future, and yet sometimes we do get clear notice of what lies ahead. I am thinking of two specific incidents that happened in that first month after Mom's stroke when she was still in the hospital. The two are more related than you might at first think.

I arrived one morning at a particularly awful time. Mom was in the midst of a massive attack of diarrhea, and it all literally hit the fan. It hit everything else as well, splattering her, the bedding, walls, floor, and equipment. She was embarrassed, furious, frustrated that no one had stayed to help her; and in that boil of emotions, she thrashed about with her arms and kicked with her left foot and sent the bedpan flying. You'd think no further damage could be done, but the bedpan landed upside down on my coat.

The temperature that January day was well below freezing, but I went home late that afternoon coatless,worried all the way about how I would cope with such events if they continued to happen. It was a needless, pointless wonder; of course it would continue to happen. The doubts I had about myself, however, were neither needless nor at all pointless; and when a few weeks later the day of her release from the hospital approached, I found that I was extremely anxious about how her inability to control such things and my queasy digestive system would mix. I expressed my severe qualms to a few members of the family, one of whom simply reacted with, "Stop whining!"

That was the second relevant event, the one I warned you might not seem related at all. It was clear to me, though, immediately clear, that a whole lot of "stuff" was coming my way and that Mom would not be the cause of all of it but all of it would smell the same. It was easy to give up the coat, but I would rather have tossed some of the family.

If you find yourself in the caregiver role, never apologize for expressing your concerns and fears. Don't refuse to ask for help. It might be safer to avoid counting on people to give it, but don't let them get too many chances to tell you that they would have helped if only you had asked. If you have someone in your circle who responds to your legitimate concerns and fears with "Stop whining!" or words to similar effect, he or she needs to cool it. I hope you redirect the fan.

~ Rehabilitation Time

One week after her stroke, Mom was ready to move into a rehab unit. She would spend three weeks there if she cooperated with the therapies her doctor thought she required. These were physical therapy, speech therapy, and occupational therapy. Her degree of cooperation varied from hour to hour, threatening her stay; but in fact she managed to hang in there for three weeks. It wasn't easy.

My sister and I accompanied her to as many of the therapy sessions as we could, a practice that met with resistance from some of the staff and a warm welcome from others. Those who were hostile said outright that they felt we must not trust them, but they were wrong. We both wanted to know what kinds of exercises to keep on doing with her; we wanted to learn the best way of transferring her from a sit to a stand. Did we need the belt that they used? How did they stand when they needed to balance her weight against theirs? What was the best way to support her when she shifted from standing up to lying down? What kinds of things did the occupational therapist want to train her to do? I did not want to go home with her and feel incompetent, needing to ask questions of everyone when I could learn quite a lot by watching. It was always a welcome surprise when any of the staff understood and appreciated our participation.

Yet in one sense we really were also overseeing their styles with her. We were upset when they spoke too fast for her to understand them and then attributed her confusion to the loss of all her abilities. She needed time to process the words, and at times they gave her more leeway than at other times. It is easy for family to fall into the trap of crossing the line between advocating for a parent's real needs and wanting the medical staff to know what a capable person this was so short a time ago. It is painful to watch the dramatic changes in ability and comprehension without wanting to assure the therapists *Yes, Mom really does know the answer to that. Here, let me tell you for her.* At one level we know that they are looking to assess her current status, and that is where they are probably right about our denial. At another level we want Mom to do well, to prove that she still has abilities. She does, and it is the medical staff's denial of that part of reality that we fight.

I wonder how much training, if any, nurses and therapists get in understanding the variety of responses they will encounter from family. Many of the staff are naturals at dealing with all kinds of people and all kinds of reactions, but more are not. Over and over, here and elsewhere, I will be asking where are the researchers in this area or that, and what are they doing? Do we need to rehabilitate the rehabilitators, or do we simply need to find ways to return to our common humanity?

~ Know Your Customer

Many issues surfaced in that time she spent in the hospital rehab ward, issues sometimes specific to her but at least as many that apply widely and that those who work in those institutional walls would do well to observe and learn from. Just as "six hundred" meant something only to me and just as my sister had reported futilely to the nurses that Mom had been fixing dinner but only two of us present knew HER, so it was, in countless situations, that we were scolded, argued with, or considered nuisances because we insisted on doing all we could to make sense of her efforts. However much professionals may know about statistical likelihoods, with rare exceptions they don't know the specific patient. Mom was so far from the norms in so many ways that it would have been more helpful to us all if the staff had been willing to observe her with us earlier or at least had stopped hampering us. She not only *seemed* to make more sense to us; she really did. They came around to seeing that she defied the usual expectations and predictions; but until they reached that point, they interfered constantly with her successes if only by denying them.

Case in point: aside from the first few days, her nonverbal communication skills – pantomime, especially – got sharper and sharper. One day she indicated by holding her hand to her ear that she wanted to make a phone call. "She does that a lot," one attendant told me; "she doesn't seem to mean anything by it." Mom repeated the gesture but could not tell me whom she might want to call. I went through the whole family, her remaining friends, her doctor, her accountant. Frustrated, she finally ran her hands through her hair and said, "Mess!" We called and made an appointment for a haircut and perm with a woman who provided such services in hospitals. Mom was very pleased. It was the uttered word that got her where she wanted to go, but she needed the gestures to make a start. I grant that nurses do not have time to keep asking questions, but that is exactly why they cannot have her answers. Similarly, they do not know enough to predict, let alone to assure family of real prognoses.

Case in point: they did not expect her to survive even six months but allowed that she could possibly make it through a year. I am sure that if anyone remembers her at all, that person assumes she died long ago. Mom recently celebrated her ninety-fifth birthday and is going strong.

Case in point: as I write in a later essay, the social worker who insisted that I was to regard Mom as an infant and not ever to allow her to make decisions and to cut off all verbal communication after dinner because Mom "had to learn" the conditions that newly prevailed. The newly prevailing conditions did not include psychological tyranny.

Case in point: they did not think she could make a single rational decision; yet she was the one who ultimately communicated her wishes with regard to the disposal of her condo and the disposition of all of her unneeded possessions. She autocratically and sanely dictated what got packed and what got trashed and who got first choice of what. Sitting in her wheelthrone, she handed out garbled orders; but repeatedly her skill at charades or pantomime got us through the hardest parts. Was it wishful thinking on our part that we could indeed make sense of her gestures and know that she still had a working mind? She not only had one; she was actively using it. She never lost the ability to let us know when we were wrong.

Often we laughed at our mutual mistakes, and plenty of times we would grind our teeth in frustration, with tears of anger and tears of sadness both. To see her in a simultaneous state of increasing dementia and valiant struggle against it, while also seeing her absolute refusal to cooperate in speech therapy, made me first admiring of her and then furious– and resulted eventually in a semiconstant battle. She felt patronized by the childlike activities speech therapy involved. "Not me," she announced; and I knew she meant that the activities were not for her but also that the way she now talked was not her.

I wanted to say to her, "Not me, either!" I am not by nature a caregiver. In this role I am not in my own true habitat or comfort zone. How could I get her to understand that fact and be less combative with me? The more her language disintegrated, the harder our daily life became. I still would not accept the judgments of the professionals, though. I knew that she was capable of more than she was letting on and that all it took to revive some of her skills was a visit from children (with whom she communicated fairly well) or some really positive excitement. Characteristic of stroke victims is the greater loss of ability to communicate when excited. Mom defied that assumption, often speaking more clearly when most upset. In fact, I once suggested giving her a tiny bit of adrenalin once a month or so because her memory, her speech, and her thinking dramatically improved when she was happily excited. Needless to say, I was scolded by her doctor for suggesting such a thing. It bothers me that we we will let a dementia patient stay locked in the confines of a damaged brain when the evidence shows that many such patients still have the content but simply need help with accessing it. Maybe adrenalin is not the answer, but something is; yet I never saw a single attempt to explore or even consider new possibilities.

One particular day, the speech therapist was working with story cards. She showed Mom a scene of kitchen devastation: a child climbing on a dangerously tipped chair, pot boiling over on the stove, water running from the sink to the floor, obstacles everywhere. She asked Mom in the tone you might use with a toddler to say words to describe the picture. Mom looked sideways at me, rolled her eyes, shook her head, turned back to the therapist, and said, "Oh-oh." Then she grinned at me to make sure I knew how seriously she took this kind of exercise. I would have loved for her to cooperate– especially in this most important of losses, communication– but I applaud her spirit and her insistence on being treated respectfully. One of the members of the hospital staff said, "I wouldn't think she'd even be aware of such things as how she is treated." Stroke did not turn her to stone!

But therein is the biggest problem with institutions. They need to be aware of the ways in which every patient is an exception to their generalities. Everyone deserves to be cared for by someone who knows him or her. Ideally, it ought to be family, in my opinion; but it cannot always be so. Institutions, and all of us, have to know the customer!

~ Blood Aunt

I wrote the following poem about my mother's older sister, but it applies to many of us and our need to have our feelings and our history respected. Of course that assumes that our feelings and history are known, doesn't it? It carries the implicit understanding that we come with diverse needs and tempers and tolerances that do not necessarily suit all those others who mean to be helpful but often have no idea of what that entails. Here is my aunt in her old age, having turned from an immaculately groomed and beautifully dressed, kind, sweet adult to the pale ghost of a near-bag woman still living in a shabby apartment alone and decrepit in every way:

I watched my aunt descend four steps:
both hands hugged the railing–
each step accomplished slowly,
her tiny body trailing
after the swollen feet.
She wants no help down.

She is ninety-three.
Her mind is failing,
her memory a shadow,
her days a slow wailing
for the friends deleted,
gone.
She has survived two men, cancer,
heart disease, loneliness slowly staling
into clammy isolation.
Offers of change are unavailing.
Firmly seated in a tiny space,
she is convinced that change will kill.

It is this inborn stubbornness
that types our blood, revealing
as nothing does more clearly
how we both are.
In separate ways we have receded;
but better a fall, a drawn-out failing,
than submit to an outside will
that knows us not.

A day came when my aunt finally did say that she needed and
wanted help, that she could no longer live alone. Some time around
her ninety-fourth birthday, she asked if she could move in with me and
Mom; but, sadly for her, I knew I could not take on more. She was
admitted to a nursing home and quickly became very happy to be there
and to be cared for daily. Unlike my mother, she made no demands.
Three weeks after admittance, she qualified for hospice care but died
within twenty-four hours. She was, all her life, a quiet woman with few
financial resources. Childless, she was unfailingly kind and loving to
her nieces and nephew. She followed her own mother's advice: make
do with what you have, and she truly meant and acted on the fact that
she did not wish to be a burden; but her final days were filled with
people taking care of her, and among her last words were these: "Now
I wish I had come here sooner."

We had tried, but none of us could force her to do what she did not want to do; and though I am sorry that she held out as long as she did, I do respect her courage and persistence in the face of extreme loneliness and finally pain. It was the pain that made the ultimate difference, the knowledge that she was dying, and the fear of dying alone. I am grateful that she was willing to change her mind, and I share her wish that she had accepted help sooner. Whether or not one agrees with her own code of values, she too has left a legacy of character and inner strength that I am glad runs in our blood.

~ Mother Tongue

Language is, like nest-building or hive-making, the universal and biologically specific activity of human beings. We engage in it communally, compulsively, and automatically. We cannot be human without it; if we were to be separated from it, our minds would die, as surely as bees lost from the hive.

"Social Talk" by Lewis Thomas

I did not grow up enjoying science or having anything more than an interest in answers to my own questions without the necessary willingness to delve into any kind of disciplined study or method. I have more the just fishin' approach to serious learning. So I am grateful to people like Lewis Thomas who bring the impossible vocabulary of the sciences into manageable portions for people like me to snack on and absorb. Their work is not only meaningful; it is free of carbohydrates and calories, yet tasty; but it is an acquired taste.

Thomas's essay, **Social Talk**, allows me to think at another level about my mother's frustration. It is easy enough to understand it at its most immediate and apparent level, that of failure to get others to understand your own meaning; but I think it has the deeper source suggested in the quote. A person who can no longer communicate naturally, successfully, and automatically loses his or her own sense of self. Perhaps it is not true for everyone who loses his ability to make himself understood, but Mom displays it literally. In her frustration she very often cries out, "I not me anymore! I not me! I not me!"

Ironically, in those heart-wrenching words, she becomes herself again. Then she will calm herself, rest a while, maybe speak a little better for a while, until she goes back to *pencil, pencil, pencil.* We understand that dementia is a dehumanizing state to be in. Sometimes, I think, we mean that the victim does not get to maintain personal dignity and that others treat him or her like an object. Bad enough! I take Thomas's thinking to mean more deeply that loss of language, loss of brain function, is literally dehumanizing by its swift and thorough larceny of our mental ability, which is what makes us who we are. What is amazing is that the brain can and does occasionally wildly scan its own inner neighborhoods and make connections again. They seem random, but are they? My mother's doctors have seemed to assume they are. It is a key question for research.

My experience with my mother has made me regret my long disinterest in science. She reminds me constantly that we still do not know any mind's true capacity; we have no idea of how much it can do in the presence of brain disease. We dismiss as incompetent people who still have that treasure chest of usable history locked inside. Someday we will know how to relieve the brain of its desperate thrashing attempts and know how to restore connections quickly.

We will need truly caring people who will take the time required to know what science will discover about us. We will learn how to keep ourselves human.

~ Weather Bird

Somehow she hears the softest rain,
the gentlest snow.
She loves to watch the sky go pink
in every sunset glow.
She notices the gradual dusk,
when pink turns into gray
and trees become mere silhouettes
at end of day.
The crickets and the birds increase.
These things bring peace.

She likes the thunder and the gloom
as much as every sunny noon.
She smiles at storms, at windfilled trees–
the tune of whose large symphonies
will penetrate her deafest ears.
They make her feel alive so much,
she wants to touch;
she reaches out
but nothing reaches back.
Then come the fears.
She does not like the cold,
no ice or sleet.

These things remind her of her years.
She huddles under covers then
to warm her feet
and warm her hands
and keep her breath invisible
and hold on to her soul.

Pixies ~ ~

I still read pepper,
I still know fax.
I look at pixies
my mother bings.
I know them all.
This one a pinic
when I eighteen;
here's my love singing
'wheatheart to me.

This a good one,
my wedding day;
he so handsome
and never gray.
Tell me, is he married now?

Here I be waiting
for second child;
she tucked inside.
I happy. I smile.
My first one grinny,
patty me.

Here all my childs
all gown up,
and here I be
with hubband two.
I 'member I lucky
but what his name?

Oh, here I be
at eighty-some.
Party for me.
Candles hum
and ev'one glow.

My first great-grand:
she cute baby.
Quick she grow,
but soon I'll see
great-grand baby
number three.

How it happen
to go right past?
My life, so fast
all gone like me.

Through the Woods and Over the River

Exactly one month after her stroke, Mom was discharged from the hospital rehabilitation center. I nervously took her home, stopping on the way for milk shakes. Start things off on a sweet note, I remember thinking. We could start our bonding by building on things we did already share: we both like chocolate.

Slowly we established certain guidelines. I gave her my room because it had its own bathroom; I slept in one of my children's former bedrooms. We brought her favorite chair from her condo, and we put it in her room. She wanted it in the living room. I said No. We had angry words or facsimiles of words. The chair stayed in her room. We agreed on dinner being at five; breakfast was whenever she awoke. Lunch was dependent on the timing of breakfast and often was just a light snack. In the beginning, she agreed to a shower three times a week and a shampoo once a week. We decided what games we both liked. We agreed that I would start getting a newspaper so that she could keep her mind working on reading. We planned menus. I learned what her favorite television programs were and introduced her to public television BritComs. Once again, despite her apparent loss of memory, the fact was that she remembered what time her programs came on and what had been happening. Thank goodness, she liked only one of the soaps.

I was happy to have her watch television for however long she wanted. I thought it would give me some free time in my studio or at my computer. She quickly realized, though, that I would disappear during her tv time, and she developed an immediate strategy. "What time?" she would call out every few minutes. "Come! What time? Where you? What time?" From this scrap of her language, you might conclude that she really had not lost all that much after all. Wrong. I am giving you the sense of what she wanted. The actual words might run more like this: "What? What pencil? Tell me pencil. Where the pencil? Tell me pencil. Where you? Come here. Where pencil?"

It took time to learn what her context was when she was making demands. She wanted me at her side at all times. Brain damage and necessity led her to invent her own words, but they drove me to have to figure out as much of her intention as possible. There were many days when doing so was just a challenging puzzle; but more often than not, her language was maddeningly generic. When one word suffices for every noun for days at a time, the caregiver's mind calls out *Enough* and begs to be excused. After all, there is just so much *pencil* a person can handle.

Being Me ~ ~

I come here now,
my mother with,
from places I not sure I me.
She not the one I always taught
would be the one who brought
me here. I did not see.
I will go home.
Here I not me.

He cook it nice, okay for while.
I stay a min or maybe week.
I way and see
where I be me.

The dark time better than I sought.
We talk, but he not unmestand.
Well, sometimes yes
but mosely no.
We see tv.
We laugh togeth.
Okay for now,
but soon I see
my home again
where I be me.

He say this home
but I know not.
I give a munce
and then I see
where I be me.

~ Aranza Panza

I don't know what "aranza panza" meant to my mother; it certainly was not a phrase I was ever able to translate with any sense of accuracy; I just know that in those early weeks together she used it a lot. The following note from my saved e-mail to friends during that time contains this paragraph:

16

I took her for a checkup Monday;
all the way to the doctor's office and all the way home, she asked
me, "Aranza panza? See the bobba dobba? Where's the lunker
doing?" but when her doctor asked her how she was doing, she
said, "Oh, I think I am doing pretty well, thank you."

Her eyes twinkled as she flirted with him, but her language really did exasperate me. In fact, I'd say that it drove me aranza panza, and I can tell you exactly what I mean: around the bend. How could she come through like that for others and make no effort to communicate intelligibly with me unless it suited her to do so? How much control did she really have? I was suspicious that she had far more in her power than anyone could guess, and I wanted her to use it for both our benefits.

The fact is, perhaps oddly enough or perhaps quite reasonably, that she never lost all the polite expressions her mother had ingrained in her from childhood. *Please, thank you, how are you? I so glad to see you, want something to eat?* None of these phrases ever was anything but crystal clear, give or take a verb or noun here and there.

I believe that that "'Oh, I think I am doing pretty well, thank you,'" goes beyond common parroted expressions; but it still fills the bill, so to speak. I cannot say, nor can my friends, that she has remained unfailingly polite. When she is miffed or angry for any reason of any size, the politeness vanishes and the language falls apart. I doubt that it really does; I think it is a weapon of hostility. It isn't as though she has all that many weapons left, and I guess I can't blame her for hanging on to what she can. I wish she could remember her own sayings from my childhood, like the one about catching more flies with honey than with vinegar. Or, if you can't say something nice, don't say anything at all. But let's face it, one of the joys and sorrows of growing up is learning that no one is perfect, especially one's parents. I hope something in her brain remembers that that applies to one's children as well. We do what we can do, and that is that. I tell myself, Aranza panza! By which in this context I mean, Deal with it!

~ Mother, Where You?

"Mother, where you?"
she asks if when she looks
she does not see,

17

if I am out of sight
or right beside her.
She has grown insecure
in this old age.

I turn the page
of photo books
and look at history.
All morning and all night
I am beside her,
despite her frequent fury
and her rage
at being so dependent.
It can't be true.

I want to run; instead I say,
"Mother, where you?
Where have you flown?
Your face how familiar
but voice now unknown,
the words all a scramble,
the intent not all clear–
but wherever you are,
I'm still here."

~ Gulls in the Fog

I am dreaming I'm at Harbor Strand,
gliding slowly above the sand.
I think it's sand.
The clouds are heavy, very low;
my circling flight is slow.
Perhaps it is not sand or cloud
I fly above, below.
It seems to me like limbo.

I hear a scream,
familiar in the dream,
familiar to my kind.
I was a solitary gull
in this dull sky,
but now another voice breaks through.

A wingtip briefly brushes mine,
although I cannot see the face
to know if this is friend or not.
I settle on a sandy spot
in a clear space
to watch the tide
and wait for fish
and wait as well for other wings.

I hear the scream again,
a second shriek, lonely, blue,
calling in gull, "Who is there?"
and "Where you?"
Where you?
I know that voice.

~ Mother, Humphrey, Dog

Over that first month after her stroke, Mom's language regressed
more and more. She seemed to lose steadily the sense of nouns and
verbs in particular– *anomie* being the condition of noun loss, but I don't
know if there is a corresponding word for verblessness. (*Averbie* is
not a term I've encountered.) And it isn't that she couldn't say nouns.
It really was a rapidly expanding case of pencil, and the problems in
communication steadily increased as frustration reached ever new
heights (or depths). As long as she had been in the rehab unit at the
hospital, I remained fairly calm and detached about the increasing
failures. Then I was not yet dealing with them alone, and it was too
soon to expect major improvement. My anxiety increased as the day of
her release came closer and closer. (See "Bad Omens".)

We managed fairly well that first day home. I was eager to make
her feel comfortable, and she was eager to be made so. I had someone
to cook for every day; she had someone who did cook for her every
day. She was astonished to learn that she liked my cooking. I was not
surprised that she was astonished. For all the compassion that I have
for her and for the situation she was in, the fact is that we had never
been close. I never felt that she knew me or wanted to know me. She
treated my work as an artist as meaningless, my friends as nonexistent,
my quiet introvert qualities as an affront to her social nature. I did not
share her values; I did not ever wish to imitate her way of life. I did not
treat her with disrespect, but I did not care to be around her. One of the
many reasons I invited her to live with me was that I had some

faint hope that perhaps we could get to know each other before the end. Better yet, what if we got to like each other? In fact, as I have said many times to many people, I hoped we could come to love each other.

So that first day, that first week even, amazingly enough that whole first month, we got along really well. Happily ignoring the social worker, we "talked" late into the night. Much of the talk was guesswork on my part, and it went on and on because of how long it might take me to make sense of her attempts; but we both enjoyed ourselves. We shared the faded blue couch and the afghan she had made and cheerfully struggled to understand each other. I know that she was happy with me; and I was feeling that I could deal with her, provided I would be getting some frequent relief.

It was partly that need of mine for getting away now and then that began to make things more difficult. She resented my leaving the room, let alone getting out of the house. I knew I could never leave her there alone; there just were too many opportunities for her to hurt herself. That assumption was confirmed one day when I had a pot of soup cooking and went outside to get the mail. In that couple of minutes, she had wheeled herself into the kitchen, stood up, and was stirring the boiling water with her hand. Clearly, it was not just her speech that had been affected; her judgment was severely impaired and would become more and more so. I worried about her trying to cook anything and burning herself, so I had to make the kitchen off-limits unless I was in there.

I knew she could fall at any moment because she would attempt to get out of her wheel chair or out of bed or off the couch with no regard for the safety measures the much detested occupational therapist kept trying to instill in her. Family members essentially were less than interested in taking her for any length of time, and hired sitters rarely wanted to return after their first stay with her. At eighty-eight, she took to cursing at people she hardly knew and who offended her with no idea that they were doing so. She also began "punishing" me for getting out, using the silent treatment– other than her orders for what she wanted for dinner. Sometimes she thought that going on a hunger strike would be more effective, but she got hungry sooner than she wanted and had to give in and eat. She "punished" the rare willing sitters in the same manner.

In good moments she called me (and everyone else) *Mother*. Her use of the word generally implied that she was feeling taken care of or at least that she had no immediate complaint in mind. The word Dog was reserved for me and never boded well. *Bitch* was not a term I had ever heard Mom use, but she conveyed exactly that when she called me *Dog*. That could be my name for several days running, and I did not respond with a smile. I just kept reminding her that I would never cooperate with her when she called me that, and I would sit stubbornly next to her saying nothing until she stopped. If that didn't work, I would leave the room for a while. On a few occasions she threatened to roll herself out the door and wait for a stranger to take better care of her. I dared her to go ahead. We were engaged in a battle for who would be in charge, and each of us was determined to be the winner. I was willing to share the power, but I wasn't going to give it all away. She reacted with that bitter glare common in people whose bluff has been called.

In fact, I suspect she knew that I would never cave in completely. On the occasional visits to my sister's house, she always returned glad to see me. I knew she had had a better time away; but as she managed to convey in clear words, "It fun, but you take better care, Humphrey." And that was the name she sometimes called me that I never figured out– Humphrey! I'd welcome any clues.

It Fun Today ~ ~

It fun today–
other mother take me to play.
This other one, she love to sing
while other other know nothing.
Today we sing old medolies
like "Tell Me What" or maybe Why?
We sing and laugh unto we cry.
She wash my hair and make it curve.
Other other do not well– not then,
not now. No how!
Today this mother love of mine
play cash with me and ha! I win.
I gab the ball and thow it back;
she give me ponts.
I win by thee.
She make us lunch;
she give ice keem;
it perfeck day
until I tired, until I pain.

Then take me home to other other,
the one who always now is mother.
She not so fun all day like one
who go with me today;

21

but when I tired, when I hurt,
she know how help.
That why I stay.

~ Alice Blue Gown

Mom's name is not Alice, but she does have a blue gown. If that statement is meaningless to you, you are either younger than I am by quite a bit or you are unfamiliar with even more old songs than I am. Anyway, when my sister and I began the hard work of moving Mom's things to my house and discarding whatever we were allowed to trash, we came upon a never-worn blue nightgown. It buttoned up at the neckline, had long sleeves, was a beautiful shade of pale sky; and we could not understand why she had left it hanging with the tags still on.

"Mine," the queen announced. "For me."

"Why haven't you ever worn it?" we asked.

"For mizzal," she said. I had a feeling I knew what she meant, and I looked at my sister. I think we both knew. "For my mizzal, " Mom repeated and folded her arms across her chest and closed her eyes. Yes, we knew.

Many times over the course of our three years, Mom would announce her impending death. Sometimes her announcement made me sad; sometimes it didn't faze me. Once in a while, I have to admit, I was ready for her to mean it. Always I accepted that at the given moment, she did mean it; and I ran up against some family anger for accepting her wishes. I never did understand that anger, and I said so. After all, we are entitled to be respected; and one way is to be believed.

There is, it seems obvious to me, a huge difference between believing a person's statements and wishes and acting to make them come true. A couple of people in the family were irate when I suggested that they needed to accept her feelings. In return, they suggested, hotly, that I should joke her out of those depressed moments, failing to understand that the last thing a depressed person wants is to be teased or to have his or her feelings written off.

And yet, as I have also learned, it can be done a little. I do believe Mom when she says she wants to die, that she is ready. I tell her that I see why she feels that way and that I do not ever blame her for having those feelings. They are normal, I insist to her, and mean it; and she smiles at me. But then I also remind her that if she does die now, she will be buried in a blue gown that has been newly ironed by her most inept daughter. Does she really want her dress creased and wrinkled for eternity? It works so often. She looks at me in mock horror, grins at me, and says, "Meb not."

The day will come when she will be past caring, and on that day I will ask someone else to iron her blue gown. It's another form of respect I will be able to give her, even if she never gets word of it.

~ Counting Games

"One, two, three, four, five," she said to her own satisfaction. "One, two, three, four, five." The first several times that she lay there on the couch counting the fingers on her left hand, I was generally relieved that she still had numbers down pat. Over the months of the first year of our joint tenancy of my house, I grew allergic to hearing the count. "One, two, three, four, five, six," she said one day; and I looked up. She still was counting the fingers on her left hand; how did she get to six? To me, it seemed a marker of a slight decline.

"Six," she proudly announced, showing me her hand, beaming as if she had on her own and with a slight hint of magic, produced the new digit. Then a bit of reality seeped back in, and she frowned. "Six?" she asked. "How I get six?" Now it was all ambiguous again, but in fact the pattern for her future was right there: progress a small amount; take backward steps; come forward a bit; slide.

We had a slew of counting games between us. She never lost her enchantment with numbers, although I must say I do not recall any such interest in her prior to the stroke, other than the previously mentioned concern with her finances. Like the Rainman, though, after her stroke, she could sight a flock of birds on the telephone wires and tell you how many there were. She could look at crumbs she had just spilled on the kitchen floor and be fascinated with how many there were. Her fascination did not prevent her from ordering me to pick up all eleven of them. Despite her self-proclaimed poor vision, she could see three tiny gnats hovering out in my studio a room away and order me to the kill.

On the other hand, I counted the hours I had to myself in the early morning and in the late evening. I counted the days until the next home visit from one of her therapists. I anticipated the number of minutes before she would throw a tantrum and refuse to cooperate.

I enjoyed the therapists' visits and so she hated them more, with one exception. She liked physical therapy, but only because she liked Stephanie herself. She cooperated only with her. I despised the home visit from the social worker who clearly knew nothing about stroke patients and still less about how to approach family caregivers.

23

Although she acknowledged that I had made the house safe, she was appalled that I allowed Mom to make any decisions at all. "Stroke victims have returned to their childhood," she explained. "You are not to allow her to make choices; you have to let her know that you are the parent now." It was another kind of counting game, and I counted the woman worthless to us. The worst thing I could have done was to deprive my mother of her reasonable rights and realistic opportunities to maintain a relationship with the person she had been. I also refused the social worker's suggestion that I abruptly stop conversations with Mom when time reached a certain hour on the clock. Who was this person, and why was she plaguing us? I refused her offer of follow-up visits, and she assured me I would be sorry. She was wrong.

Hospital personnel had had their own counting games. They had warned us that whatever progress Mom made by the end of one year, presuming she lived that long, would be the farthest she would go. Somehow, in some bizarre imagining of their own or that of the experts whose work they studied, 365 days was the magic number. Mom had that long to show her stuff. Today, seven-and-a-half years later, she is still making progress. At ninety-five, having survived the stroke, a fall that resulted in spinal fusion surgery, over a hundred benign falls, a two-week bout of pneumonia, Mom still astonishes us with sudden recall of complex sentence structure, bursts of memory, and intelligent questions about her own status. Also days of complete unintelligibility, total confusion as to where she is, loss of names of the family (but never her own), and an overall decline in her personal hygiene. She has re-remembered most details pertaining directly to her– although she thinks at times that the 22nd of every month is her birthday and gets briefly hurt if we aren't celebrating it. And on many days she also forgets all those things that she knew a day before or five minutes ago.

She has an amazingly accurate sense of how many friends or relatives have come to visit her and how long it has been between visits. She recognizes all faces, despite the absence of names. Some days all that matters is what she has lost; other days what matters is how much she has retained. She counts so many things to pass the time: fingers are her favorite; bruises to her fragile skin are another. There are always the crumbs and the birds and the number of consecutive days she has demanded a bagel. Sometimes counting is just a rote activity that she remembers she has done; sometimes it is a way of relieving a bit of her boredom. She never expected to find herself in the unhappy state that she is in– for one thing, her self-esteem was always strong and still is. She has always believed in her worth and dismissed those who criticized her. Even so, she has on occasion wondered if she would ever matter to me; but if she did doubt me before, I believe that she deep down knows it now: I see how much *she* counts.

~ So Smart, So Stupid

Stupid was another of the red flag labels she had for me, but not only me. Others were stupid if they thought she did not understand them, really stupid if they patronized her. She would patronize them in return but share her disgust with me after they left. This pattern annoyed me a lot since others all felt that she was eternally loving and that my criticisms of her were unfair and petty. I knew who of the two of us was the pettier one, and it was the person who dismissed everyone who did not immediately gratify her wishes.

To her, I was stupid if I did not understand which of the thousands of meanings of "pencil" she was using. I was stupid if I didn't know the answer to her routine question, "Where is the . . . ?" While the formula part of the question was always clear, the noun that followed never was. "Where is the horse? Where is the diggery? Where is the mother? Where is the dog? Where is the pencil? Where is your husband?" While the first five of those were at least not emotionally charged, except maybe the one about Dog, the last one was often said in a tone of malice. After all, she had not approved of my divorce some fourteen years earlier and let me know quite often that it was an embarrassment to her. I could not feel sorry for her on that score. Her constant value was on the appearance of things and on the pretended denial of reality, and mine has always been the opposite in most areas.

Occasionally, though, I was not stupid at all. When she knew that her speech was especially unclear but that I had succeeded nevertheless in understanding her, she would beam and say, "We so smart!" She not only said it; she meant it. One of the things I consistently got praise for was my ability to decode her pantomimes. One of my favorites, but definitely not the hardest, came before we sold her condo when she was trying to tell me the location of some item in her dresser still in the condo. First she had to distinguish between the chest of drawers and the triple dresser itself. She did so by making two rectangles with her hands, one wide, the other narrow. "This one," she said, repeating the wide shape.

"Not the chest of drawers," I said, "the dresser." She smiled very happily. Then she pointed to the left and said, "Iddle. You know iddle?"

"Little. The little drawers on the left," I said. More smiles. Then she pointed to the right and repeated, "Iddle." Yes, I knew she meant the little drawers on the right. Then she pointed to a spot between the two extremes and proudly instructed me: "Biddle! See? Biddle-biddle."

I knew that Lewis Carroll would have been proud of her for so creative a portmanteau: she had successfully led me to go search in the middle big middle drawer, where I subsequently found exactly what she wanted. That day we were oh so smart!

~ E.T., Stay off the Phone!

One of the early puzzles that never went away was Mom's voice. Only rarely was it the voice we had always known; mostly it became an outer expression of an entirely changed person. Whereas it had generally had a pleasant quality, it became harsh and extremely nasal. It was as if she had forgotten how to use her vocal equipment and was struggling to relearn technique– not struggling anywhere near enough, though. It also took on a very childish whine, not endearing. It was most irritating when she was refusing to hear or cooperate, and those times seemed to come more and more often as we moved past the three-month honeymoon phase. In some ways she began to sound like the alien character, E.T.; but it was only amusing when she would sing with my sister *Let Me Call You Sweetheart,* always a favorite.

This voice problem, combined with her language impairment, made phone use very difficult for her and for others. It was an exercise in major teeth-gnashing, and I had to be the one who tried to interpret each side to the other. Few could understand her, and she could not usually hear the other person or process the words quickly enough to understand what was being said. Still, she did enjoy getting calls and claimed to enjoy making them. I had more than doubts.

Her statement that she had called this person or that person was one more way to tell me that I was not necessary. "I talk to Pencil. I call Pencil today," she might say. "He say he glad to tell me. I sing Pencil for long time. For hour."

"Which Pencil did you call? How is he or she?"

"See, you know nothing. Nothing! I call peep evday."

Well, I knew she had not called anyone successfully. I knew that even if she had located her address book and had found the correct numbers, she could not have reached anyone. I knew what she did not know, that our area codes had just changed and she would have had to dial three extra numbers she had no awareness of in order to call anyone she knew. Sometimes I am oh-so-smart even when she thinks I know nothing at all. Sometimes I am positively knowledgeable!

Once in a while she would ask me to dial someone for her and would make me leave the room. Did she really think that one wall away she was inaudible? Yes, that is what she thought. She invariably was looking for someone to rescue her from the extreme pain of not getting her way in all things. Aranza panza. Ironically, she always had to call me to be interpreter.

I think it all would have bothered me a whole lot less if she had used that maddening E.T. voice when speaking to most of the rest of the world or, better yet, had lost that voice quality entirely.

~ Shopping with Grandma God

In that first year, she liked to get out of the house. We visited friends of hers; we visited her two older sisters; we would go get milkshakes; we ran short errands. We went out for dinner sometimes, with or without others. What she liked best was to go to the grocery store and steer the electric shopping cart. The good thing about the cart was that it gave her a sense of control, as if she were once again in the driver's seat in every way; the bad thing was that it really did give her control, and she drove it at its slow-fixed pace steadily into display cases and on a couple of occasions into shoppers. Only once did she get caught in a spin that she could not get out of for a minute. Fortunately, she enjoyed the ride. It exhilarated her, and her speech briefly improved. "I like that," she said cheerily and clearly in her normal voice.

There were other bad things about shopping together. She somehow became absolutely fixed on the idea that the stores she had formerly shopped at were now no good, and she would develop one of her tantrums if I headed toward one of them. The local discount food chain was OUT; Walgreen's had offended her in some obscure way; and although I have no idea what these stores had done to lose her as a customer, I mean that she was THROUGH with them. On one trip, she ordered me five miles out of my way just to avoid buying a birthday card at the nearby drugstore.

The topic of birthday cards reminds me of one card she had ready to sign and send to one of her grandchildren. I handed her a pen and some scrap paper to practice on. She ignored the paper and painstakingly, slowly, deliberately, scrawled GRANDMA GOD. Personally, I thought it reflected her genuine feeling about herself, a self I was not worshipping. Still, it was in these things amusing and peculiar that she built the best memories I have of our time together, just as one of my favorite childhood memories of her is of a time late at night, after we children had gone to bed. We were awakened by a strange sound downstairs in the hall or kitchen. As if it were Christmas and we spying on Santa, my brother and I silently crept down the steps. Mom sailed by, wearing my roller skates and my skating skirt that could not come close to being able to be closed around her waist, and waving Hi to us. When she is in a good mood, she is always fun and always was.

There were other good things about shopping together. She could make quite a few decisions at the store. She could feel that she was teaching me how to pick out cantaloupe. She could let me know that buying certain items would be a total waste of money, because her face revealed every feeling. A smile was always a good sign, but she was also adept at pantomiming a gag. Subtlety was never one of her arts.

~ Sundowner's

I don't think I was aware of the Sundowner syndrome before Mom came to live with me. The name has a poetic ring to it, but the reality has nothing of romance about it. When the sun went down and the moon came out (or not), Mom didn't become a werewolf or anything of the sort; what she became was more fearful and confused. Previously a nightowl and always one to stay to the end of a party, she now filled with anxiety and became obsessed with getting home as soon as twilight struck. Then, all the way home, she would cry that we were lost, that she had "nev seen any this pencil afore." She would scold and nag every foot of the way, unless she decided to close her eyes and try to doze. I wished she would do that each time we were out.

One beautiful summer evening, a friend and I went to a nearby driving range to hit golf balls; and Mom was happy to go along. She sat in a protected area and watched, calling out occasionally, "Oh, that a big lunker," for a relatively decent shot, or smiling at each of us if we even just made contact with the ball. When we finished, I noticed that I needed to get gas for the car and drove to a nearby filling station. Her reaction was swift and loud, bitterly denouncing the whole idea and angrily insisting that we get home immediately. She was furious and it wasn't even dark yet. In her normal days, she would have been far more worried about the possibility of being stranded in the car without gasoline. That thought surprisingly seemed never to enter her mind.

I'd like to know what specific things get triggered in that mind. Does her vision diminish more than ever in the lower light and scare her? What causes the panic? What language is she speaking inside her head? It is pointless to tell her that everything is fine, because to her it isn't fine at all. It is definitely frightening.

One night we went to meet my sister and brother-in-law for dinner, and I drove one block past my turn when traffic prevented me from getting in the right lane. The moment she realized that I was turning around to reverse direction, she began insisting that we go home right away, that I had no idea what I was doing, that I was endangering us both. I wish I remembered how she conveyed much of that, but she succeeded. When we arrived at the restaurant a mere five minutes later than planned, she announced that we had been lost and she had been "so fightened."

Sundowner's can be far more extreme than the version Mom had; but it still became mighty inconvenient that first year when we were getting out a lot. I never missed it later. I suppose things might have been more interesting if she *had* turned into a werewolf; but then I'd be writing an entirely different book, if I could write at all.

~ Seasons

~ i ~

Winter comes, a quiet time.
The world seems sleeping now.
Covered up is all the grime
and thick the walkways all with snow;
the light is low.

Strokes come and fill
her brain with gray,
seeping content at their will
to unknown places far away.
Night runs into day.

I watch my mother fight
at first; she seems so tame
and sweet and bright
when nurses, strangers, ask her name.
She thinks they're playing some new game.

Reality sets in: deflation.
Her life was outer motion.

~ ii ~

Spring comes, dissipating rime
and reason too. She's sleeping now.
In days when she was in her prime
she'd still allow

her mornings to start slow.

Back then her afternoons would fill–
errands run at height of day,
grocery shopping, paying bills.
"You have to work before you play,"
she liked to say.

I hold fast to a different thought,
that work and play must be the same.
Whatever art is or is not,
work has to be a joyous game
to satisfy its highest name,

re-creation.
My life has been reflection.

~ iii ~

Summer comes aghast.
Her therapy's just work, not fun.
She notes green leaves are holding on,
but "ello" is her word for sun.
She wakes at one.

Now she is focused on her age
and plays the helpless soul.
Often she goes into a rage
at minor things– a stocking hole,
an unremembered mole
that she has counted every day.

I watch from windows old and new,
and see her through my blinds.
The daughter gets the same old view,
but silently the caregiver finds
that stroke affects at least two minds.

Depression.
Past from present is estranged.

~ iv ~

Evening, autumnal, comes at last.

Her therapists are long since gone.
All her life is in the past;
she thinks that she's the only one
whose span is nearly run.

She trusts that life lives on one page,
her own experience the whole
of what is good. She speaks,
an incoherent sage,
as if society must extol
the way she's played her role.

I cannot think her way is true;
I know it binds
and keeps us small. I grew
along a path that winds
away from her. My role I knew
would be expression,
but one swift lightning stroke
and my world changed.

~ Serpent Teeth

How sharper than a serpent's tooth it is to have a thankless child.

King Lear, *William Shakespeare*

    I admire Shakespeare's Cordelia in her steadfast refusal to be
bribed into her father's excessive demands. In many ways I also
identify with her. Lear was a needy old man; and had he been a decent
listener and a king who knew his daughters and his subjects, he would
have had all he wanted and probably a whole lot more. Instead, he
went by a rigid literal interpretation of statements with no regard for
truth. I think the only reason for the play's sake that Shakespeare made
him a king is so that he could have a Fool handy to mock his ways.
Ordinary citizens lack such luxuries and would have to manufacture
their own inner Fool, but how many have the time or real inclination?
    In her long healthy years, my mother ruled in her queendom and
would have been horrified to think that she would ever need to be
dependent. One of her mantras used to be, "I don't ever want to be a
burden to anyone." She meant it, but life does have its grim habit of
contradicting us. Long before the need, I had told her that if she ever
felt the desire to stop living alone, she was welcome to move in with

31

me on the condition that she not need constant nursing level care. At the time she thought that was very reasonable and so did I. From the earliest weeks that she did move in, it was all too clear that Mom had no further problem being a burden.

Looking back, I would say that although there were many little things that she demanded right away, the biggest change for the worse came after three months. That was when we both encountered all the stress and work of clearing out her condo and moving all of her possessions. Some family members did pitch in and help quite a lot; others did not. For me, the end of that work did not come with moving her out of her former residence– that was just the beginning. No matter how much we threw or gave away, there seemed to be more and more stuff generating descendants in the dark closets. It all showed up in full force in my already crowded house, and way too much of it is still here.

The sharpest bite of the serpent's tooth comes when Mom in her extensive ability to be a burden has a sudden increase in public intelligibility and loudly and coherently screams at me, "You do nothing for me!" The accusation took on a slightly comic twist one time. We had been to a family party, a bridal shower. Her great-nephew, the groom-to-be, freshly in from California for this event, came over and kissed her on the cheek. "He do more for me than you ever do," she later told me. So I sat down and made a partial list.

<u>Much of what I do</u>

I cook all your meals and eat with you.
I shop for and with you.
I help you do laundry.
I bathe you and wash and set your hair.
I help you with your therapies.
I take you to all appointments.
I make sure you visit others.
I arrange for them to visit you.
I talk with you and play games you like.
I make sure you take the proper meds at the right times.
I try to keep you from harm.
I clean up after you.
I clean YOU up after you.
I take you for wheelchair rides in the neighborhood.
I encourage you to try new activities.
I listen to you and make every effort to understand.
I keep track of all your paperwork.
I write most of your thank you notes.
I keep family and friends informed about you.

I try to make you smile and laugh.
I accept that you still want to live and that you also want to die.
I reminisce with you and share photos to help you remember.
I take you on small outings for variety.

I have given you my daily life, but you are Queen Lear.

<u>All of what he does</u>

He kissed you– and, by the way, so do I.

Yes, my patience can be exhausted.

~ Patience (an occasional virtue)

Ordinarily I have a fairly high patience level. Anything whose
delay I can understand, I can accept, even though my preference is for
immediate resolution to all problems and instantaneous satisfactory
closure to all situations. I don't like unanswered phone calls or
unanswered mail; but if necessary, I can respond to the same question a
multitude of times despite hating repetition. There just are times when
repetition is going to happen. . . and happen. . . and happen.

It is not unusual for my mother to ask me what day it is as many
as thirty times in ten minutes. "What today?" And I can calmly say
Monday or whatever day it is every single time. She can ask the
time more often in a minute than you'd think possible. "It's nine o'
clock." I might give that answer fifteen times before I have to say,
"it's one minute after nine." I have assumed that she simply needs
to communicate and that time is the topic of the moment. A healthy
person asking would drive me crazy.

When it comes to insults, I have no patience at all. One *you stupid*
is grounds for an alert: "If you call me that again, I'm leaving the
room." Here at home, if there was a repetition, I would head for my
studio. I have learned to exit mentally or bodily in other situations
with other people– not that a whole lot of folks in my life are given to
insulting me, though there is at least one. On the phone or in person,
it's goodbye. People will say what they want to say, but no one is
required to listen.

The difficulty with a mentally disabled parent is that all the old
conventions are constantly tested. I was taught early (and accepted as
natural) the need to respect my elders. I have generally found that easy
to do; but respect, like patience, can meet its limits. I expect respect

33

to be mutual; and when it isn't, mine dwindles. It is rare for me to be deliberately rude, although I have heard myself say at various times in my life some things that I had no intention of saying and for which I still privately atone– but not one of those things was ever addressed to my parents. The rule of respect held firm and still does. Respect and patience, however, are not one and the same.

I suppose that what I value now is reasonable patience. I try to stay easygoing about the things that are inevitable or at least that are unalterable, but I don't have to be equally calm about any excessive demands and ridiculous assumptions. I can choose to be patient if it helps the situation and an angry crusader when rights get trampled. Sometimes nothing matters but expressing anger. Patience becomes one more demand and often more than one too many at that. That's when I have to remind myself that is only an occasional virtue, and that's just fine with me.

~ You Call Me Cold

What makes a child fall to earth?
What skins her knees?
What chills a child in the sun?
The sight of foxes in the fields?
Taunting? Teasing? All of these
and more.

Were I not born a child unmade to please,
I'd dance for you or sing your tune
or both of these
and more;
and you would call me warm.
But I was made for quiet arts
and hide within my sleeves.
My heart's my own, my thoughts, my deeds,
and my beliefs,
and more.

You want a song that I can't sing,
a dance I cannot do.
No matter what I can provide,
my gifts are crumbs to you.

Were I designed like squirrels

to scale the rough-ridged trees,
I'd build a nest with those I love
or play alone
or both of these,
beyond the reach
of you and more.
I'd seek the thinnest branches,
build with the thickest leaves.
I'd hide secure from foxes
in my house beneath green eaves,
my castle in green air.
Taunts might not reach me there.
I'd woo night winds to rock it,
dream to a tidal breeze,
or nap my soul in sunlight,
all of these
and more.

But now that you are frightened
by the way that you've grown old,
I find I'm tangled in your vines,
to keep you safe from harm
while others go their distant ways;
and yet if they just say hello,
and that is all,
you call them warm.
So who is cold?

~ A Thing of Beauty

She pokes my arm
as if she were Hansel's witch
testing for plumpness to eat her fill.
I shrink, scabbed,
touched by the almost dead,
contaminated by her tissue-paper skin,
refusing to be gingerbread
for her to nibble on.
Where is the love I should have for her?

She seems to do no harm,
but her ways are such as kill.

Sooner, later, I too have had my fill.
Today this is not love I feel for her.

We are grown crabbed
by one another, led
by rosy notions now exterminated,
the myths on which we've fed,
that mothers' love and daughters' love
are reliably, inevitably
a joy forever.
A daughter's a daughter for all of her life,
a plural-edged knife,
sweet-sounding only on one crumbling surface.

I try to rise above the stubbornness
of both our angers; it is wrong when she is sick,
I say, and how could I sever this tie?
There is danger in this self-talk,
filled with guilt from blinded others
who say loved ones cannot be a burden,
especially mothers,
anointed by fable to saints.

But this protracted tending is not always love,
nor any form thereof;
it is tyranny double-jointed
to a lie.

~ Guilt From Association

I don't know which is the harder guilt to deal with– that put
unfairly on you by others who do not know who you are and what you
are dealing with or that put squarely on yourself because you do know
who you are and what you are dealing with. For me it was usually
easier to ignore the guilt trips that came from outside. In the first place,
they came from people who were refusing to participate in my mother's
care or who had no rightful role to play at all. In the second place,
their real goal seemed to be to make sure that I would not trouble any
of them with the burden of knowing that all was not rose-toned delight.
Some of her grandchildren operated under the delusion that Grandma
was a generous all-loving sweetie. It's one thing to love and appreciate
your grandmother and quite another to glue her to a pedestal

and keep her there no matter what facts come along to tip her over. Let's be honest: Grandma was a self-centered purchaser of affection who did make large gestures but who expected specific compensation. She modeled a range of little values from extreme pettiness to outright undermining in her pursuit of her own interests. She had two widely disparate selves and could switch between them at the slightest flickering of disagreement.

All that said, she also had amazing strengths— extraordinary tenacity and resilience, profound practicality, a kind of common sense mixed with a disinterest in logic that sometimes worked against her, and a devotion to certain aspects of family. So, even here, I am hedging on her strengths. Her tenacity about having her own way in the lives of others was always very annoying, even insulting; yet quite clearly her tenacity has helped her survive in this long, perhaps too long, life. Her resilience has allowed her to overcome fatal odds repeatedly and to cope with and survive the pain and deaths from cancer of her two husbands. Like tenacity, her practical nature also contributed to her ability to cope with those challenges that life presented to her. Positive and negative equally mingle in these strengths. Her common sense led her to make wise purchases, to provide food and shelter for her husband and children twice over. All this is good.

When it comes to nurturing, I have to distinguish between at least two different kinds. Yes, she provided food, clothing, and shelter. During our younger years, Mom provided plentiful food that lacked flavor or chewability. She sewed a lot, but clothing she made tended to come apart at the seams. We didn't mind this as much as the food problem. We had a house that was heated and had furniture, but the furniture was an aesthetic nightmare. In a way, I think I do admire that she was not so concerned with appearances in that area, but she was overly concerned in so many other ways that I didn't understand why we had to be subjected to horrible color combinations and ugly design. The future artist in me stayed permanently repelled and added to my horror back when she tried to insist that her things oust mine.

More importantly, she did not know how to nurture emotionally or, at times, even physically; and so the house was a home only at times. Excellent at entertaining family and friends, she all too often ignored the needs of her children. Examples? For one, she let my sister stay ill for almost a month before getting her to a doctor, who immediately recognized rheumatic fever. I remember some of the great-aunts hovering at a family gathering, upset that my mother was dismissing the complaints as a cold. They knew it sounded like rheumatic fever and finally told her so. That was when she agreed to consult the physician.

Other items: she allowed my brother to be bullied harshly by our father, who had a swift and hot temper. She simply denied that there was anything unusual in the pattern before her eyes. Later she would deny that it ever happened at all. I was a child, and I knew that fathers should not shove and threaten and hit their children, not for large matters and not for small ones.

In my childhood, she showed no concern about a major change in me from sunny little extravert to very fearful introvert. I was going through daily torment from around-the corner neighbors; and all she ever said was, "You've become such a crybaby!" In my fear, I never told her why; but when I had children of my own, I had to wonder how she could have just let it go. Clearly she had noticed the difference.

My fears and nightmares did not make it easy for me to make friends as a child. Her way of dealing with that problem was to tell me how much it hurt her that she had a very unpopular child. She would say this repeatedly, pointing out that she had many friends. Could I appreciate her concern? Not at all.

So it was very interesting to me to learn after she moved in with me that some of those many lifelong friends wanted to let me know that I was taking in a very difficult person who did not "deserve" such care and that I should reconsider what I was doing. Family might be in denial, but her friends were not. Oddly, one of them seemed to think that she was sharing a fact previously unknown to me, that my mother had never really liked me, that she would refer to me as the black sheep. Did they think I had been blind to her behavior all my life? Apparently they did. And can I understand how a quiet, well-behaved, cooperative daughter who never got in trouble and was an honor student (who had even made friendships) could be a black sheep? Her comment confirmed in my own heart and mind that we had little to say to each other. If I had to be her clone in order to be loved, I was willing to forego the love and to accept the consequences. I just never understood back then why she needed me to be like her. She seemed happy enough with who she was.

But it has been of equal interest to me to see how my mother dealt with learning that I do have quite a few friends– a fact she was not happy to learn at all. She was hostile to some of them, indifferent to some, jealous of every one of them. My friends visited; only a couple of hers did, and those two did not come often enough to suit her.

Do I feel sad about acknowledging and sharing these ugly, unkind realities? I am sad that they *are* realities. Do I feel guilty about this acknowledgment and sharing of them? No. Do I feel guilty about the quality of care I provided for her? I have no reason to feel so. Am I without guilt in any way? I have a strong sense of compassion for all victims, certainly including my mother; but love between us has come slowly and erratically and painfully. For many years we rejected each other while acting as if we did not. For that, I share the responsibility with her, and I am sorry for both of us; but another of my many reasons for offering to be her caregiver has been that I did not want to go on rejecting. It was an act of atonement on my part, whether she was able to reciprocate it or not.

About a year ago, the doctor and nurses and I all did think she was about to succeed in dying. She was enrolled in hospice care because she had stopped eating, had stopped getting out of bed. She folded her arms across her chest and closed her eyes, waiting. Every so often she would open one eye just a narrow bit to see if I was still sitting there and would smile kind of slyly when she saw me. Once she found me with tears slowly rolling down both cheeks as I sat there watching her trying to will herself to death. It was a both sad scene and a silly one. However, she reached both arms out to me to gather me in for a warm hug, and she smiled the most incredibly beautiful smile I had ever seen on her face. She finally had me where she had always wanted me: lovingly sympathetic to her and melodramatically returning to the sheepfold to honor her soon-to-be dying self. She was so pleased that she perked right up and began eating and wanting to get out of bed. Within a week or so she was the picture of wrinkled health and was evicted from hospice when evaluation time came around. Once again, her resilience and strength had overcome depression and self-pity, but I have to admit that her resilience and strength can often deplete my own.

~ The Genie Is Out but not about

I enjoy thinking that if I were granted three wishes, I could spend one of them on wishing for several more. I hope I would not make the mistake of wishing for an endless stream of genies, because I feel sure that all of them would come with dead batteries. Used up. Helpless. I'd probably have to feed them. I'm sure they'd need a bath.

I'm willing to have specialist genies. My art genie would guarantee me a prominent place in art collections around the world and enable all of my descendants to go to good colleges. First, my children have to produce a descendant or two or more. My writing genie would guarantee publication of those writings I really want published and would ensure great reviews. I don't expect to meet those magical figures any time soon, not in my lifetime. If I do, those putative descendants might reap a few more benefits.

It is the caregiver's genie who is on my mind right now. The things I wish for in this context are really possible. They are not dependent on the caregiver working hard enough, skillfully enough, luckily enough. They are things that ought to be the right of all caregivers.

First, I would wish that every one of them (us) had the full support of family and friends. By full support I mean intelligent emotional underpinning, NOT undermining. I mean significant relief for reasonable lengths of time. I mean adequate compensation in ways specific to the needs of the individual caregiver. Maybe it is financial; maybe it is in household help. Maybe it is in meals provided or in means to have personal care. It will not be the same for all. These are human needs, and it does not require the mythical and magical to make them possible.

Second, I would wish that caregivers be given tax benefits. Those of us who relieve the government of huge Medicare and Medicaid payouts and do not ask for welfare could still use some kind of consideration in the form of keeping a little more of what income we still have. A lower tax rate might enable more individuals to have the financial wherewithal to consider becoming care providers for a parent.

Third, I would wish that those who criticize us for not doing what they would do– or for doing what they won't or can't do– would keep their opinions from us. We are the only ones who know what we need to do, no one else. Don't accuse us of false motives; don't even assume you know what they are. Don't tell us how to proceed or when to stop. You don't really know.

But then, if I could have one truly fantastic wish, I would ask that none of us ever need genies. I would hope in some utopian way to discover a world where people do not suffer devastating damage and intolerable grief. We could live our lives to our human strengths, not forced to confront human weaknesses and flaws and disintegration. The genie is out, not out of the lamp or the bottle. Just out. Perhaps to lunch, although I am feeding none at the moment.

I have a theoretical interest in human magic. I use the word as a catchall for all that we do not presently understand but that transforms, and I don't expect that we will ever be without such mysteries that confound our minds and senses. I regard all forms of healing as magical; I regard deep friendship as wondrously magical. I am in awe of specific genius that sees possibility where most of us see merely confusion. I admire logic but do not believe it is enough to solve all mystery or to bring us to our true selves.

Given these feelings, I am not stepping out of character to daydream about genies. Somewhere in the universe there is a container of answers, abstract or concrete– maybe kryptonite, maybe glass, maybe a cosmic brass lamp. Whatever it is in a material sense or whatever it is in a spiritual sense, it is the holder of the knowledge we have yet to gain. There are folks who think it is wrong to seek that container. They might cite Eve or they might refer us to Bluebeard's ill-fated wives as cautionary tales about probing too far. I believe, though, that we are destined to explore all things, to move beyond all barriers, to look within and to look far out in our efforts to know not only ourselves but our true origins and our true human destiny. Let the genie out of that vast container, and let us shatter our limitations. As long as there is intractable pain in the world, unbearable grief, unaccountable greed, blissfully deliberate ignorance, overwhelming power in the hands of any, we will never achieve freedom.

Bring on the genies without the tricks, the ones who reside in the spiritual jars, the ones who grant not just wishes but true answers. Then let us hope that we do not stone them.

~ Something to Remember Him By

I have said that I had many reasons for taking on the role of caregiver, including my wish to atone for my part in the coolness that existed between my mother and me almost all of my life. Probably equally important to me was to counteract some of the memory of my father's final conversation with me. I had grown up loving this Prince Valiant of a man– the epitome of the tall, dark, handsome, silent type (except when he was angry). I hated his temper bursts, but I was very rarely on the receiving end of them. I identified with his love of sports and his creative energies, and his values in countless ways became my own. He liked what he called the natural look, and so I wore no other makeup but lipstick. He was more interested in doing than in reading; I was interested in both. He came from a lower-middle working class family, and my politics arose from his rarely stated but definitely Democratic views. He was a wonderful father to a little girl in most ways, though certainly not all. An absolute perfectionist, he settled for nothing less even when we were small. A job done poorly was a job about to be redone. A job done well was a job that always could be improved with practice. In some things I am a perfectionist, but not in any of his ways.

I remember with total clarity my task when I was three, when our family moved to a house. He set me on top of his workbench, poured out thousands of washers, bolts, nuts, screws, and assorted nails from bags and boxes. He gave me lots of clean, empty baby food jars and ordered me to sort every single one of them by size and shape into the jars. It was not difficult, and in fact, I loved doing it; but not every three-year-old will sit patiently and sort them flawlessly no matter how long it might take. That was my assignment; and years later, when my mother finally moved out of the house, those jars still contained those perfectly sorted bits of hardware. I have none of his orderliness

41

or level of demand on others, but I do have some of his overbearing obsessiveness about small matters.

It took me many years to realize that the value he held for naturalness did not find any takers in our family but me. My mother was always made up when she left the house, as is my sister generally. Hair styles changed at whim for them; mine stayed pretty much the same– one long version and one short. I got rid of the long version over forty years ago and never went back to it. It took me even longer to consider that his reason for such a value had nothing to do really with thinking that people looked better as they were and a whole lot more to do with how much better-looking he was. I think he wanted to keep it that way. After all these years, I hold onto the value while having little respect for what I think was his real motive.

He was not quite the same great dad when I reached my teens. Another of his values was learning by being thrown into the deep end, literally and metaphorically. Just as it was true in the swimming pool, it was also true in social situations; and on more than one occasion I was left stranded late at night when he had assured me he was picking me up from some social function but never came. Most of the time he did; but now and then he failed to show up, and I was left to walk home alone in the dark, angry and worried and frightened. I felt that he did it intentionally, and I was increasingly upset with him. He, in turn, just became more difficult to be with.

It is very hard to know how long his cancer had been developing and how much a part it played in his changed behavior from towering Prince to little man. What I do know is that in his final moments with me, four days before his death, he asked me to help him get rid of his pain. I was eighteen and back then only morphine could relieve his pain. Or death. No matter how much I wanted to, I certainly could not. "Then get out of here and don't come back," he said in a hoarse whisper. "You are useless to me, and no man will ever love you."

I went home stunned, with a severe earache that lasted exactly four days.

o o o

I don't know if I am lovable or not to men like him, men who think a woman's only place is at their side or at their feet, devoted only to their wellbeing. Quite bluntly, I cannot say now that I find men like him all that lovable myself. Love and need go two ways. Sometimes I imagine encountering him in a dreamlike state and running in the opposite direction. Sometimes I imagine rushing into his arms but never to ask for his forgiveness for not being able to rescue him from pain and death. I find that I love him in spite of his words, but I have been thoroughly hurt by them. Sometimes I expect him to apologize, but most times I don't.

My mother, not knowing of that last interaction, thought that I did not go back to the hospital because I was too weak to bear to see him dying. The truth was that I couldn't bear to hear him. Over forty-five years later, having never fully recovered from the blow to heart and mind of his words, I saw my mother in great need and whispered hoarsely to his shadow but equally to my own, "Whether you love me or not, I am not useless."

~ Applefall

What made me so susceptible to slights?
Each day I hang– an apple on the tree,
grounded, bruised. Then come bewildered nights.
I rise on branches every dawn
to fall again,
not knowing what is needed
to end the psychic storms
and end the bleak eternal *how?*
How do I find my way?

No simple thing to say because one writes
that one must always keep the bruises fresh,
that even when the world,
the tree, make clear their lack of heeding,
that one may never loosen grip on thorns
but always mortify the soul's own flesh
and go on bleeding.
All who are crucified for who they be
participate in mystery.
No Christs are we, no hounded Eves,
though we too hang on apple trees
and feel through pain
and see from banishments
life's stark indifference.
No complex thing to say because one writes
that what we feel and what we see
become our life and history.
And if the world and tree revolve
around, away, from each of us,
and all of us devolve
to dust or ash,
what matters whether joy or pain

be ours, so that we find our truths
ourselves
on our own boughs?

~ Don't Bank on It

Hospitals and the world of medical professionals in general are not the only places to encounter institutional intimidation. Banks have techniques all their own. I thought we were ahead of the game since Mom had wisely set up a living will, a living trust, powers of attorney for health and financial directives, successor trustees. She had been in her own mind an exemplary role model for minimizing the burdens on her children in the event of her illness or death. It was incredibly disturbing, therefore, to see what hoops institutions can roll into your path in the name of security.

I had that power of attorney for her medically and financially. In addition, my name is on her checking account and her safe deposit box. I am her Disability Trustee and legally entitled to act in her behalf and for her benefit. Imagine my surprise to be told that the bank had no legal responsibility to honor any of it. The choice to do so or not was entirely in their power. Do attorneys know this and simply withhold the information? Bank representatives insisted that I bring her in to sign a document stating that she was capable of making the decision to allow me to take over disbursement of her funds. "My name is already on all your documents, and she signed them when she was competent to make such a decision. Now she isn't and that's why she created the trust in the first place," I had to repeat to countless managers, assistant managers, personal bank representatives, tellers, and a few people whose titles I never caught. They seemed to transfer to other branches on a weekly basis, so I rarely saw the same person twice.

"We are not obligated to honor those documents," they all stiffly replied. "She has to come in."

"She is not able to walk or to sign her name," I said. "Would you accept 'Grandma God' as a legal signature?"

Banking personnel seem to be required to leave their senses of humor at home or in the parking lot. "This is a serious matter," they uniformly responded.

"Yes, it is," I agreed. "To whom do I report your total lack of cooperation? You have copies of all the legal documents, including statements from two attending physicians that she is no longer mentally competent, and both of us have been customers here for a number of years. This is not personal banking at its best, despite your advertising slogan."

"We are under no obligation to keep the copies of her papers,"
they said. What? Why not? I didn't get it then, and I still don't. Their
policies were keeping me from being able to pay her bills, were making
frequent trips to the bank an onerous necessity, and were as totally
obstructionist as possible. At first, they also challenged my right to go
to the safe deposit box, but my name was indelibly there on their rolls.
It was a long fight, and finally I did gain access to everything. It is
nice to know that they care about security, but who will protect us from
them?

~ and Blue

I remember her smiles, laughter,
her energetic rush
and push to action and event,
not forgetting her small deeds
inside their large façades,
gleam applied to bland,
crass, petty,
but once in a while something
genuinely grand.

Now comes a hush
beneath her white bone rafter,
stroke-sent. In concrete ways
present she is, not yet hereafter.
I mark the date when days
turned into decades, sand
refused to fall in the funneling glass.
The sundial stayed in shade.

I see the cinders of her mind,
her centric thoughts charred sparrows
that think they still are larks
or poisoned arrows, verbal darts.
Highly she esteems her power,
though jabs are quivering fluff,
pale down, unlettered,
in this ember hour.
Were they ever really not?

My rush of daylight fire
is banked in the ashes of her halting night.
What will quicken the dead,
infuse, inspire,
make my life right
demands her life instead.
In every sense I wait,

yielding to the caregiver's guilt:
willing to serve what's right,
devoted to what feels true,
yet wanting a life of my own,
a dream not on hold,
unfettered,
rising beyond the barricades
and soaring Gold
and Blue.

~ Bonus Time

My mother had generally had some kind of household help, even
in the days she and my father could barely afford it. I never had, and
I had felt embarrassed at the thought. It is that democratic ideal that
one person should not do the work that another doesn't want to do.
Fortunately for those who want or need such work, not everyone feels
the same. The woman who had been coming to Mom once a week was
willing to shift her operations to my house, and that provided me with
enough time to make those idiotic banking trips or make short trips for
extras at the grocery store or even to sneak into forbidden places like
Walgreen's or discount stores.

It worked out well in other ways, too. Mom felt that she had a
friend coming in, and she really did; but it was also good for both of
us that once a week someone else would clean her room and keep the
kitchen floor clear of obstacles like a wastebasket or the table clear of
newspapers. I was never good at housekeeping, and Pat made a huge
and wonderful difference. For one thing, she talked with Mom, who
enjoyed the new voice. What I did not like is that Pat's presence gave
some family members that much more reason to feel no need to visit
Mom on any kind of regular basis. It bothered Mom a lot more than it
bothered me, except in the respect that she was unable to believe that
they might not want to visit and so chose to accuse me of deliberately
keeping them from seeing her. She had no idea how willing I was for

anyone and everyone to visit her as often as they wanted. Neither did they, or maybe they did but just didn't care.

It would be pleasant I guess to think that they presumed that I was doing a good job, but I don't make that assumption. Before Mom did move in, I had asked my brother and sister each to contribute at least two days of care per month. That pattern was never to materialize, and I still have some resentment about it. Even Mom knew that their response was wrong, except when she wanted to blame me. She reminded me that she had shared the caregiver role for her mother with both of her sisters. Each one tended Grandma one month out of three, and no one felt overly imposed on. I think she is right that these responsibilities ought to be a shared proposition. As it was, I burned out after thirty-three months, and they never got to know their real mother. Their image of her is what they want to remember, not what it is. When one of my nieces said that she didn't want to remember her grandmother the way she was now, I was upset with her. To my way of thinking, the greatest gift you can give those you love or those you want to love– or just say you love– is to accompany them to whatever their future holds for them and to accept them as they are in every present moment. You don't allow your mind to stop them in their tracks and not allow them to make new ones. I think that knowing the real her is a bonus they opted out of and one that eventually, slowly, painfully I would come to appreciate far beyond my expectations. It took a long time, but our relationship did grow.

~ It's Funderwool, It's Marblous

Despite the geometrically increased difficulties of living with someone whose communication skills are totally capricious, there is also the humor side. I recommend enjoying it as much as possible, letting sensitivity be one's guide. Mom laughed at many of her mistakes and tolerated others' laughter up to a specific point: do not patronize her! Do not laugh at her, only with her. If she was amused, we could be. If she was not, our laughter rightly made her angry. That is a boundary to respect.

Some of her word concoctions were wonderful. You could see how she got to them and even credit her with logic, not usually the case– e.g., *biddle*. Some were reversals of syllables; some were near misses; a few were so appropriate that they should have gone into Webster's Unabridged Dictionary immediately. The best put us into hysterical fits of giggling, from which she would briefly surface and say, "What that mean?" and then return to the giggles, like the time she announced that her onion hurt. We looked at each other and simultaneously raised our eyebrows and opened our eyes wide and got giddy. "What I mean?" and that set us off again. (No, it wasn't a bunion.)

She'd come to breakfast announcing she "feeling kinda chunky." Not fat, hungry. She would roll herself to bed, waving like the Queen Mum, announcing, "I go squeak now." When surprised, she'd look up and shake her head, saying "I be darn!" And when I did not translate successfully and made a silly face to let her know I didn't get it, she would laugh but say precisely, "You look stupid." It was futile to ask how insults could be so clear and everything else so fuzzy, if stated at all. Her language was, to borrow a family phrase, a puzzlement to us all. Sometimes it was a Pandora's Box, storing things you wouldn't want to hear; sometimes it was a little treasure chest of chuckles.

It seemed so obvious to me that she should be the one in charge of our expressed reactions to her, but I was surprised and hurt for her that not everyone who visited felt that way. Some insisted on laughing at every mistake, and she was deeply offended. There isn't a single rule about acceptable reactions; but if you let the situation and the person guide you, it isn't all that difficult to know where the lines get drawn. Just pay attention to what seems to cause her pain and what seems funderwool to her. And be grateful for every scrap of humor, because each one is marblous.

~ Stand and Deliver

In addition to her language and judgment impairment, Mom had lost considerable strength down her whole right side. She could not stand or balance herself and essentially required a wheelchair to have any mobility at all. The day she was released from the hospital, she came home with her brand-new chair, and it was to become both a necessity and a nuisance for both of us. She came home with walker and cane as well, but for a long time she had no interest in them.

The chair was one of the smaller models but still awkward and heavy for me to lift into and out of the car. It was never easy to get her into or out of it either. She would try to get up from it, frequently unlocking the brakes no matter how many times the therapists would try to make her understand the need to keep them locked when she wasn't moving along in it; and she would lose her balance. She eventually became adept at turning corners to get from room to room, but the paint on the walls was soon chipped and scraped from her early narrow turns. The relatively new carpeting steadily acquired dingy ruts. It had taken me a long time to earn the money to buy that carpeting, and I grew very depressed just looking at it. It seemed to be a matter of indifference to her.

Gradually, very gradually, physical therapy made a significant improvement in her strength. She developed a secret plan. It would have been impossible for anyone to guess as much. She continued her stubborn opposition to other therapies; she appeared ever more helpless and demanding. She had been mildly cooperative at first about trying a few activities– knitting, reading the newspaper, occasionally playing the piano, playing a variety of games, and working puzzles. She never did lose interest in games, but the other activities slowly vanished. I struck a deal with her about the piano: I was getting no exercise at all (and hate to do it– I preferred sports but had no outlets), but I told her that I would do exercises as long as she accompanied me on the piano. Up until that offer, she would play for a minute or two and want to stop. With a malicious grin, she began playing longer and longer until I was the one who put an end to the arrangement. She was very pleased with herself.

I think it was sometime in the late autumn, although I really no longer remember things by dates, that I was working on the computer and heard an unfamiliar sound. I did not hear wheels moving along the wood floor; I heard footsteps. I literally bounded out of my chair to go look for her, when into the living room she walked. No chair. No walker. No cane. Lurching a bit drunkenly and with her hands dangerously inside her robe pockets, her face lit up and beaming, she made her way to me and delivered herself into my waiting arms! "Look at you! Look at you!" I said, laughing with tears flowing a bit. "Wow, look at you!" We stood and swayed together in a sedate little dance of joy. Suddenly she was happily exhausted, but she walked into the kitchen and I fixed a celebration breakfast.

We both stayed in wonderful moods all day long, both genuinely pleased and proud of her; and yet it was a whole new worry. Those hands in the pockets scared me, and she never stopped putting them there. It gave her a sense of security, while giving me the opposite feeling. For several weeks she happily wobbled around the house, happily demonstrating her amazing progress to every visitor. We never told anyone; we let others learn the same way I had. A guest would arrive, and Mom would suddenly walk into the room to the startled face and the beaming smiles of approval. She never tired of it.

She did, however, nearly kill herself.

Look Me ~ ~

Look me, look me
I standing, see?
I make– surprise!–
this long journey.

Along the walls
I creep so slow
and where I go?
I do not know.

I look for Mother,
her I show
what I can do now all alone.
I go home now.

I ready now. I me again.
I walk, I talk,
what more I need?

She there, she smile,
she laugh with me;
we dance together,
one, two, three.
But now I tired as can be.
I go home soon.
I me! I me!

~ Another Reason, Another Season
(forget the whoopee)

    I guess I should apologize to the ghost of Eddie Cantor, who
sang the song alluded to in the title. I'm not even sure how you spell
"whoopee" as he sang it, and my context here is entirely different from
that of his song. Nevertheless, it seems like a good title for a piece on
additional reasons for becoming a caregiver. I did say that there were
many.

    I had been living alone for a number of years at that point; my
children were all adults scattered around the country; I was feeling
almost as useless as my father had said I was; and I was finding myself
burned out in painting. There was nothing I wanted to write. I felt

isolated and mistakenly thought that taking care of Mom would in a way also take a little care of my own needs, especially the need to be needed.

Among the many things I learned was that being over-needed was debilitating and mind-numbing. There is a very thick line between being needed and being abused. There is nothing vague about that line; it is not there in the sand; it is embedded in solid ground. It fossilizes and refuses to budge. But what is "over-needed"? How do we define that thick line?

In my personal dictionary, it is a normal need for a person with dementia to rely on a caregiver for all the routine daily requirements–making meals, overseeing medications, doing laundry, assisting with whatever help with personal hygiene is required, providing transportation to essential services and to social functions, participating in conversation every day, and other essentials that crop up. It is most definitely not a normal need to require the caregiver's constant attention and presence every moment of the wakeful day. The problem is, how does one succeed in conveying that message to someone whose brain has lost much of its reasoning capability and even more of its short term memory?

That thick line also separates genuine loss of ability from the manipulative, convenient loss of ability. Here the problem is knowing what the truth is, but truth's content is a whole lot blurrier than that solid line. I needed a way to know, but I never found a reliable one. It is impossible to measure loss that fluctuates constantly.

Just now, a cardinal has landed at the feeder outside my window, and now it is gone. That is how Mom's memory is, and that is how her ability level flits from place to place. One moment she is grounded, and the next moment her language and thought have flown away. If I could have been beside her every moment, reinforcing the skills she sometimes has, more of her abilities might have returned. It is a level of need beyond my capacity to provide. It is over-need, and it is deadly to the caregiver's soul.

~ I'm a Lumberjack, Yes I Am

Over the years, I have watched relatively little television, and lawyer shows are a big reason that I turn the tv off. I've listened to the sharp clever dialogue and the alleged analytical skills that prove that by every logical reason, Mr. So-and-So had the motive, the means, and the method to do in either Mrs. So-and-So or her wannabe replacement. Juries are shown seriously pondering the logical proofs, but we all know that logic has very little to do with human reactions. I present this point of view for very self-serving reasons that seem funny to me, but what would a lawyer have made of the circumstances?

We had had a very heavy thunderstorm one night, and we awoke to tree limbs down and branches dangling and debris scattered throughout the area. It happened to be a day for Pat to come and clean, and I took advantage of my short time off to get to a hardware store where I purchased a small chain saw to cut the fallen limbs into logs and to trim the dangling branches and twigs from the tree trunk. I did not give it much thought; I just went and got one.

The night before, Mom and I had had one of our spats over whether or not leftovers were suitable for the Queen; but I wasn't thinking of that when I examined various sizes and weights of saws. I knew I needed a lightweight one that I could hold, and that is all I was considering. The dawn of awareness came when I returned home and Mom's eyes opened very, v e r y W I D E. She stared at me, at the saw, and a look of deep fear took over.

Now, I will grant that at that moment I could be said to have had a motive. I clearly held a means and method. The fact that I have never wanted to harm anyone suddenly seemed frighteningly unprovable. By sheer lawyer logic I could have been convicted on the spot, except that there was no crime. Nevertheless, I spent a sleepless night trying to prove to an imaginary judge and jury that I bought that chain saw for the branches, which I did. I have used it many times in the past several years now; and while Mom still bleeds easily and does often look as if someone really has attacked her, she does so in the relative safety of the nursing home, just as she did in the more questionable safety of the hospital and in the best safety I could provide at home.

Once she knew how I used the saw, she would get herself to the living room window and smile and even applaud my performance. I don't think she ever had imagined her daughter, whom she had trouble understanding all our mutual lives, would become a lumberjack. The thought tickled her, which, it seems obvious to me, is not the logical effect of chain saws. I'd like to rest my case.

It is essentially a question not of logic or clever lawyering but of personal morality. The old saw of a different kind, *the thought is equal to the deed*, is so blatantly false as to be insulting, not to mention extremely dangerous. Human imagination will produce an endless chain of thoughts, images, fears, possibilities, dreams, nightmares, alternatives. They serve us well much of the time, allowing us to prepare for contingencies. It is what we do once those images rise to consciousness that matters. Does everyone who gets angry become a murderer? Does every parent who gets frustrated with a child's behaviors become an abuser? Should every thought be subject to inquisition?

What makes all the difference is how we deal with temptations of the spirit. Do we yield to every impulse however fleeting? Or do we understand that we are subject to anger and disappointment and frustration and exhaustion– and that our inner imaginer is far more fertile than it often needs to be? Do we have the power and the will to override it when it goes beyond the boundaries? Most of us do. Whether we do so out of a fear of punishment or a love of life and civility, we choose to be moral. Without such deliberate choices, morality is a meaningless word. It is freedom of choice that creates good and evil, morality and immorality. Our reasons may vary widely, but the choices we make with our freedom are what come forth to characterize us.

On the day I brought my purchase home, two people had a chain saw reaction. The fear in my mother's eyes struck me in mine. Her frightened expression made me even more aware of how much power she realized I had over her, and my real actions subsequently reflected who I am– a person with a developed conscience built not from fear of punishment but from respect for life and with a need to cut branches but not from the family tree.

~ Playland

They ask me why I do not take
you to care centers for my sake,
but my sake is the point.
Do you remember Playland?
You took me there
when I was three
or four so you'd be free
to shop without a clinging child.
I sobbed and screamed all three long hours,
locked in the bad children's cage.
They told you I'd been *very* bad–
poor tactic, for it made you mad.
You knew I was so mild.

I have not forgotten Playland.
For once, you took my side
and without asking why I cried
promised we would never come again.
We never did in all the million hours.
Now would I do to you

what you could not be brought to do?
Would I place you where you do not want to be
so I could be for hours a bit more free?
Should I drop you at a lecture you cannot hear?
Should I dismiss your anger, ignore your fear?
What would be the point?
I would be forgetting Playland.

Oh, there may come a day
when I will have to override this vow
to care for you
and for important reasons
that don't exist right now
may have to say Goodbye.
We both may have to cry.

Not now.

~ Why?

I remember having many past conversations with a friend who insisted that guilt is a useless emotion. I have never agreed with that, but I do think that asking *Why?* about major life events is a useless question unless you are willing to accept an answer. Why do some people seem so uniformly lucky? Why do some people attract wealth? Why are some people in pain all their lives? Why any tragedy at all? Religions have developed to deal with the questions, but none offers authoritative answers for all.

I am not willing or able to believe that anyone is immune to pain and suffering. If pain is a possibility for anyone, it is a possibility for everyone. It does not have to imply punishment; it reflects the reality of bodily existence. We are not built for physical immortality, and there seems to be an infinite variety of ways that nature has of doing us in at last. Worse, though, are the many ways we have of doing ourselves and others in, accidentally or intentionally. In this explosive age of terror rocking the world every day, we look in vain for answers to the questions, *Why war? Why killing? Why hatred?* In this high speed society we learn to our unending grief that there are very drastic consequences for a moment's wrong decision.

In the narrow world that my mother and I inhabited together, the question was far more personal. Over and over again she would ask,

"Why this happen to *me*?" The answer is, simply, conditions were ripe for it. God is not punishing her; her own body reacted to its own biology and chemistry, and the result was a stroke. Naturally this answer did not suit her.

I think of one of my uncles, a healthy man all his life until at the age of ninety-two, he learned that he had leukemia. He could not believe ill health could come to him; after all, didn't he love his wife (and her cooking, as he seemed to think was relevant)? He genuinely acknowledged that he had had a wonderful life; therefore, God, why are you threatening it now? Why ruin a good thing? His eyes filled with tears each time he reflected on the fact that even he could die. It was incomprehensible. Mortality belonged to others.

Mom's attitude was slightly different. She accepted that such things could happen, but she wanted to know why she had to go on living if she could no longer be who she was. To me, it is a much more poignant question. My own response to her was that at the very least she was a terrific example of strength and resilience and that she was leaving her descendants with quite a legacy of character. She would look at me, dismiss all that as nonsense, and say, "What about ME? Why I here for ME?"

That egocentricity is another side of her legacy, the one I hope not to inherit. I already have my fears, though. I really have my doubts.

~ Bird News

It is a morning for the birds,
hunger being rampant
and the feeders being full.
Brilliant little yellow
and duller olive finches,
pinky purple ones with stripy mates,
tiny chickadees and sparrows
jab their tiny beaks
into the plastic gates to get the seed
from every perch.
I keep on adding feeders
to the branches of the cypress
so my mother can enjoy them.

Quite a brunch gets made midmorning,
till the cardinals and blue jays
swoop down to claim their bigger rights.

Then, all heavy flutter, the doves
land from their favorite roost, south gutter,
to scavenge fallen seed
down on the ground.
They've forgotten how to search for food
at any height and simply go around
in cooing circles, pecking stones
there in the mud or on the concrete driveway.

At noon my mother rises fully dressed
to observe them,
but the frenzy is all over.
Small and large, they all have scattered
to some new or old address
and left her where she does not want to be.
Still she stands there by the window,
hoping they will soon return.
Quietly she calls them but no answer.
Finally she eats and naps.
She has forgotten what her daily pattern was,
thinks the day is merely eating time,
thinks dark clouds mean night.
So she rests her eyes, her bones,
in little patterns of her own
that slowly wear away her days.
In sleep she can forget the things
she can no longer see
or dwell among them should she choose.
No longer has she any use for schedules,
though nature does.
By early evening all the starlings
come settling from the tops of trees,
from the cypress and the oaks,
from the sweet gum decked in burgundy
and yellow leaves.
Lordly iridescent blokes
who think nothing of their brothers
but whose intelligence is higher than a dove's,
they attack the plastic feeders from above,
knocking seed in careless wingswipes
to the dying grass.
They harass the meeker, smaller souls
in their haste to reap the seed.
They strut like little generals

and instigate small wars; they seem to think
to do so is their proper role.
Later, Mother slowly wakens
to the fact that it is dimmer,
almost dark, no longer summer;
and again there are no birds in sight.
It wasn't summer earlier at noon,
but she's forgotten that.
Somehow she does remember dinner
so I go prepare her meal.
Like the doves, she knows she's hungry
but waits for others to provide.
I scavenge for a little for myself.

It is a narrow day
with windows narrower yet,
too small to see the world,
although I don't forget, not being just a bird,
how I prefer to search at many heights,
not choosing like the doves to poke the earth
and merely wait and hope.
Oh, I often peck at stone, at sand,
but not at them alone.
I'll seek dessert among the stars
in and out of constellations
where consolations linger
in those distant tiny lights,
in among the largest starlings
where there's eternal possibility
of cosmic wings
dispensing manna freely
to all who hunger for it.

~ Can I Help?

It's a question often asked and too often left unanswered. I'd like
to tell you that Yes, you can help. There are many, many ways.

Right off the bat, I would suggest if you are the friend or especially
the relative of a caregiver for a member of the family and you are
unhappy with how that person is handling things that by all means you
take your concerns directly to that caregiver. It isn't discussing and
disagreeing and coming to new conclusions that is upsetting; it all

has to do with how the disagreement is handled. Please do not storm in and angrily express your views. Stay polite, calm, civil, and ask your questions in a tone of genuine concern. *Genuine* matters. Before you express disagreement, find out how each of you views the whole situation. You may be angry that your parent isn't showering daily; the caregiver may be struggling to get Mom or Dad to bathe even once a week. Safety takes priority over spectacular hygiene; and if the care receiver is uncooperative, there is fear– the bathroom is one of the worst places for falls.

You may think the caregiver has made all the decisions; find out how much is a necessary compromise with the care recipient to have any kind of peaceful relationship. You may have in mind all kinds of improvements in arrangements; first learn if they suit the parties most directly involved. Find out why things are set up as they are. Then, if desirable, make your suggestions.

You might think more outings would help everyone; are you offering to be the person who takes Grandpa on that outing? Perhaps you think the caregiver has signed on for a one hundred percent time commitment to be with Grandma for the rest of their lives. Keep silent on that one because it's an outrageous expectation, but go ahead and make opportunities to provide relief for hours or days at a time. Don't pile guilt trips on the person who is doing the work.

You can offer to bring in groceries, whether you or the caregiver pays for them. Or you can stay with Dad and let the one who tends him get out alone or with friends. You could invite one or both of the twosome out or to your house for dinner occasionally.

The age-old advice holds true: put yourself in the other person's place. I have learned a number of things about love and compassion; and of the two, I think compassion is more helpful and also more enduring. The more compassionate and empathetic you become, the more you want to do what helps, and the more you realize that you feel that way about life itself, not just those close to you. Love may want to accomplish the same goals; but often it becomes maudlin, so personally sentimental that it may fail to be helpful at all.

You want to help? Try to imagine yourself in the role and ask yourself what you would want. It's not an impossible task.

~ Lifeline

I have lost count of the number of people who have commented on what a blessing we have in our long-lived family. In many ways they are right. I grew up knowing all of my grandparents, one great-grandparent, many great-aunts and uncles. The women in my mother's family tend toward extremes, either dying way too young or way too old. Mom's mother died at ninety-eight, mentally alert, physically in great pain from spinal cancer until her doctor found the right dosage of medications for her; her own mother died in her early forties. Grandma was the matriarch of the family; all loved and honored her. Her three daughters had none of her mental acuity in their final years. The oldest, presented in "Blood Aunt," stayed fairly alert and active until about ninety when her last and best friend died. From then on, her mind and memory steadily declined until the point when she had virtually no short-term memory at all. She survived by notes to herself all over her tiny apartment– notes with phone numbers and notes to remind her of where she kept more notes. Her survival was minimal, though. It would be truer to say she existed– in the same clothing and eating the same frozen meals– each long and lonely day. Her life was not, for her, a blessing but a curse. Occasional visitors made her briefly happy, until she forgot they were there and took herself off for a nap.

The second sister also remained active until a bad fall made walking extremely painful. She too continued into her nineties to do housework and drive dangerously to all her errands and social activities and to cook for that very appreciative husband who thought that death portended an end to home-cooked meals. And I assume it did mean that. After his death, my aunt developed more and more problems, both physically and mentally. She did not lose all of her memory as her older sister had; she did not have a stroke as her younger sister did. She simply developed a dementia all her own, speaking clearly and intelligibly but with no reality. If she was in bed, she might ask to be put in bed. If she was sitting in a chair, she might want to know why people were keeping her in bed when she wanted to be in a chair. I don't know if she was hallucinating being where she wasn't or if other things were going on that we had no way to understand. She, too, died at ninety-four, a miserable woman and one in great pain. I can't call her long life a blessing. On the other hand, one great-aunt was still enjoying driving from California to New York and back alone at ninety-six.

My mother has always been a very competitive woman. I privately believe that she has stayed alive despite herself because she wants to be the one who lives the longest. If true, we have at least three more years of increasing debilities, probable falls, small strokes, anger, bitterness, and frustration to live through and very little compensating pleasure. Somehow I doubt that it will have been truly worth it to her just for the post mortem pleasure of saying, "I outlived you all!"

~ Our Cross

I listen to the locusts stripping all the trees
while a steamy summer breeze with no volition
hisses at the window where my mother sleeps,
snoring like a hornet cluster
and feeding on gray dreams.
Nothing protects her from nature's fierce invasions,
though her ears are partly deaf
and like the windows close
against life's muffled murmur.
It still is there, just within her ken.

Someday not all the sizzling of the bees
will wake her; not all the rounds of ammunition
wasps can wage or birdsong drop upon her deeps
of sleep will irritate or fluster
or penetrate her stony self
or matter or incite. It will take teams
of angels with tantalizing visions
of lost loves and fully blooming roses
to stir her.
And what then?

Here at the feet of aging trees
once climbed to freedom and vocation,
I see my own loves wither on the branch.
What angel keeps them safe
for days when I might muster
strength and passion for what always seems
my eyes' and heart's ambition?
I am a kind of Moses,
journeying toward a promise,
sure that it exists for some;
but then again
I see the lumpy body on the bed,
the atrophying arms and legs
below the burnt-out head.
We sojourn in a wasteland, dregs
of what we were
but still one small step short of dead.

She floats, a horizontal line.
From where I am, I look at her,

at where she lies and what she was,
at what she has become,
while I stand in her presence
vertical
and dumb.

~ Not a Rose

Not everyone is a rose. If I were to assign my mother a flower name, I think it would have to be Cactus; and I don't mean that in only the negative ways. The more I consider it, the truer it seems to me.

Without doubt she is a spiky personality, uniquely shaped by her experience and by the conditions of her life. She has been formed by the suns of her loves and the winds of her sorrows into a tough survivor who thinks highly of herself and her competence. She stands her ground, whether it is in the bedrock of her beliefs or the sands of quirky fortune.

Born to loving parents who were able to provide a secure, though not wealthy, home, she grew up confident that she deserved whatever she could afford, whether that was a lot or a little. She accepted both situations and learned how to accommodate the wide variations in circumstances. When the sun scorched, she always had rain stored for need. She was quintessentially pragmatic.

Knowing these traits, I find it hard to understand why she was not a more sensitive parent herself. She loved very unevenly and very narrowly, no matter what words she used to describe herself. She saw herself as a model of generosity and lovingkindness, while many saw her as cold and self-centered. She was a mix of both extremes. In the midst of plenty, she was unfailingly generous with gifts. In the heart of her children's pain, she had nothing of substance to offer. She modeled the petty and superficial and suggested the worst alternatives. She raised her daughters to avoid experience and to live in fear. Her daughters do not thank her for such gifts.

I've been asked if our relationship was always a love/hate one, and the answer is No. It rarely reached either level. I respected her in various ways but did not like her. Yet she is who she is and it is true that has always had every right to be so. No blast of wind has moved her from her core; and I applaud her for such strength of character, whether I like the person she is or not. Until recently, I did not. It really is only now, in this relatively empty time of her long life, that I can admire the flower that is blooming in the desert, this tough cactus.

~ Make of It What You Will

I dreamed one morning that I was walking with a friend through a sunny field. We were talking quietly, but I could feel myself getting more and more exhausted. I continued walking, slipping increasingly into a daze, and suddenly felt alone. I turned to see my friend far in the distance, surrounded by children in that sunny space, but I continued forward. Each step became more difficult, as if I were being pulled into the earth by quicksand. I saw a flight of steps that seemed to lead to a cool porch. Each step was slow and sluggish, each more difficult than the last. I felt the air around me shift, felt that the air itself was growing dizzy. The scene in the field blurred slightly.

I heard my friend call out to ask if I was all right. I could not answer. "Are you okay?" she called again, but I had no voice. I wondered why she asked. "Sammie is there beside you," she called in a worried voice.

"Her dog Sammie died," I vaguely remembered. "Have I?" But my friend could see me, and I could see her. I could hear the children laughing in the sun and see them dancing in a straggling circle. I could not stay to watch them, and I turned there on the porch and went through the double doors of a large stone building. I have been to that building in dreams before and know that its corridors go on and on forever. I had no strength to walk them, and so I rose into the air and flew. The ceilings were so high and the walls so dark and cold. It managed to feel like both a cave and an enormous prison. I knew a way out and flew straight through the walls, into a whole new space.

If only it is like this, I thought. A leap into and through all barriers, into a whole new space.

~ Next Step on the Journey

The time came when I could no longer take care of my mother. Even if I had not had two serious falls, it would have been time. She had become increasingly incontinent and unwilling to allow me to protect the bedding or couch, as well as increasingly difficult to help get to her feet or to bathe. She stopped wanting all the personal care other than shampoos and scalp massages because everywhere else she was hypersensitive to touch. Her skin could bleed profusely from the slightest contact with a washcloth. Her limbs were bruised from the small act of putting her arm down on a table or having the back of her calf rub against a chair. The merest breeze would chill and hurt her. Everything was too much effort. Her heart and lungs, though, were extremely strong.

I had decided that I would continue taking care of her for a few more months, that I would make the final decision to move her after we had celebrated three full years together. We liked whole numbers. But the first of my falls came as a result of stepping on a wet spot on the kitchen floor where, unbeknownst to me, a few ice cubes had fallen and melted. I slid through it like a first-time skater and went wildly sprawling across the floor, a platter of meat just out of the oven in my hands. In an effort to keep from burning myself with the hot food, I threw my arms outward. Not only did I fail to prevent myself from being badly burned; I also tore apart my right rotator cuff. I could not raise my arm at all, nor could I lift anything much heavier than a paper towel. I couldn't reach anything on an upper shelf; I could not bathe her or wash her hair or my own.

I managed to go on for about a week or more by asking my sister to come bathe Mom, by using only dishes and utensils in lower cabinets and shelves, and by calling on friends and neighbors when neither Mom nor I could manage some specific situations. It was not good.

Then I fell the second time, tripping over a raised area of sidewalk that was covered up by leaves. I went down in a flat in-your-face kind of fall, and then I knew I had really done the shoulder in all the way. I had surgery on it a few days later, right after we moved Mom into a nursing home. I thought briefly that she would come home again when I recovered. Six weeks later, when my shoulder was fairly well healed, I knew I could not bear the thought of continuing as caregiver. I applied for a job, knowing I needed to be with other people, with adults who could communicate, with people who did not keep me on an emotional roller coaster. I had found some salvation for my mind during my time with Mom through the use of my computer, and I was lucky enough to get a job at age sixty as a computer specialist in one of our local schools. It was a lifesaving move, and the timing was perfect. There is no place like an elementary school for kind appreciation. I crashed through the home walls to find myself in a whole new space.

Strangers and Other Neighbors

The transition from home care to permanent institutional care is a difficult one for all concerned. It is less traumatic for respite situations or other temporary needs; but, like it or not, accept it or not, the goal of final care is by definition the move toward death. One need not be there long, whether as resident or as visitor, to realize how much death permeates the entire place. Walls may be decorated; cheery music may be playing somewhere; games may be going on in one area or another; staff members may be smiling; administrators may be incapable of saying the word "resident" without putting the word "dear" first– but one trip down the hall with drooling residents half hanging out of their wheelchairs or staring into space or screaming obscenities will wipe out the thought that you have entered or crossed into anything but the final frontier. The welcoming lobby and the main dining room may be attractive and clean and filled with the most competent residents; but the living areas, the bedrooms and bathrooms, will tell a different story. It is not one to read as a bedtime treat.

Sad to say, but all too often the living areas smell of human excrement; the aides are rougher in the privacy of bedrooms; the kindness of some is defeated by the indifference of others; the costs are exorbitant and frequently erroneously billed. I say this about even the self-proclaimed high quality facility Mom entered. Look beyond the initial appearances, and you will have material for endless guilt.

What was hardest for my own mother was being surrounded by residents who seemed to her to be far less capable and farther into their own private worlds than she ever became. She was right about the private worlds, but her judgment about competence was fairly thoroughly skewed in her own favor. She was no more competent to live alone, though she thought she was, than any of the others she looked upon with disdain. A naturally gregarious person, at first she attempted to communicate with the more intelligible people she encountered; but they avoided her. She stopped speaking to any of the many people who became, one after another, her roommates. She did continue off and on to be friendly to a few of her neighbors there, but put two language-impaired people together and you will most likely get very frustrating conversations at best. If they are not overwhelmingly depressing, you can hope that they will at least be entertaining. For Mom, choosing between sitting with the others in the hall, close to the nurses' station, or staying in the loneliness of her own room was easy. Most of the time she chose her room and sleeping. Not until she was confined to bed after a fall that immobilized her for several weeks did she want nothing to do with her bedroom. She condescended to sit with the others, generally counting her fingers or dozing. She became one of them, and the transformation was very painful to observe.

My sister and I would go and play games with her– bingo, cards, dominoes, anything for which she could remember the rules and play– although I stopped playing a few games because she also remembered how to cheat. My sister would sing to and with her. We both would bring in photo albums and new pictures of family members. All of these things were tolerable but for only so long. She always wanted to go home.

The first year there, we took her out to eat on a regular basis; but that too came to an end. As she became increasingly unable to control bladder and bowels, she decided that she did not wish to risk public embarrassment and told us not to take her out anymore. We had family parties in the nursing home on special occasions, and she loved those; but she still wanted to go home.

For some, life in a nursing home is an improvement over what their existence had been. Certainly that was true for my aunt. For others, its main function seems to be to make one willing to face death, soon! For those of us still on the exterior of the Home, life there becomes unbearable to contemplate, even when we realize and foresee running out of other options. Community planners, I ask you also, *Where You?*

~ Another Old Saw

How often have we all heard the expression, *truth is stranger than fiction?* I have a collection of stories I wrote (and still add to) that deal with two quirky women trying to accommodate their later middle-age years by sharing a home and working somewhat together. Some of the stories are serious but many are outright farce. I learn from both kinds, and one of the things that I have repeatedly learned is that I probably should never expect anyone to be able to live with me again. Shades of my father's curse! But it isn't likability or lovability that is the issue or question in these stories. Caring about another is always present, but daily life is quite a complicated thing when very different personalities and very different needs share a common space. The collection was my foray into imagining what it would be like to share a life and a place with someone else again, this time on a completely different footing from marriage. I was not anticipating being a caregiver; I was mentally exploring a possibility to see if I could, even in imagination only, live on an equal basis in a companionable way with anyone.

The point I am moving toward is that in one of the stories that was intended to be totally satirical, I have one of the characters pay a visit to a nursing home. The other, worried about the meaning of this trip to such a facility, goes looking for her and encounters the absurd, one of my favorite topics. I wrote the story long before Mom moved in with me, let alone moved into a nursing home. What I have discovered to my both pleased and horrified surprise is that my story was absolutely realistic, nothing truly farcical about it. I'd like to include it here.

The collection of stories is called *A Herring Sampler*, and you probably need to know a tiny bit about the two women. One is an artist and writer– who could that be?– and the other is a most excellent community citizen, organized for committee work and for genuine acts of kindness and caring but with just as keen a sense of the absurd as the other. They go by the superficially wacky names of Sniffle and Nosemitt. Don't be put off, please, by those names. The women are a bit odd but not fools. Logic and the ridiculous coexist in both of them.

~ ~ THE HAVENCLEFT KIPPER CAPER

> *kipper: v.t.; to cure (herring, salmon, etc.) by*
> *cleaning, salting, and drying or smoking*
> *- Webster's New Twentieth Century Dictionary Unabridged*

step one: baiting and catching

"The time has come," Sniffle announced somberly.
"I'll bite," Nosemitt said; "time for what?"

step two: a brief cleaning

"To visit the Home." Sniffle went off to her room to shower and change out of her paint-spotted jeans into something less comfortable, something suitable for scouting the Home. Nosemitt, still on pause in the kitchen with the newspaper motionless in front of her face, allowed the phrase to seep in. Then, after due consideration, she got up, went to the foot of the steps, looked up, and said nothing. She shook her head and went back to the paper. She changed her mind and began to clean up in the kitchen. It was going to be another of those days.

step three: a prologue and then the admittedly metaphorical salting

Fifteen minutes later, Sniffle was back in her studio counting the number of framed paintings hanging on the walls or stacked against them. "Twenty-six," she reported to Nosemitt and left. Again after several moments' delay, Nosemitt went to the back door and stared at the garage. Perhaps Sniffle was planning to pay her way into the Home with paintings. It wouldn't work of course, but what else could she be thinking? *Why?* was another question entirely, one that for the present was unanswerable. Nosemitt debated, got her purse, checked for keys, and went slowly out to her car. The only Home Sniffle might qualify for, the only one they had ever discussed as a distant future possibility, the only one that took apparently healthy and fully ambulatory citizens still in their fifties, was Sunset Tyme Retirement Center. The two of them referred to it as Last Resort and could only speak of it in joking terms, but it was the only one Sniffle could mean.

Its parking lot was small and practically empty. One blue pickup truck was in the shade of the only tree; one very rusted and beat up ex-hotrod had been deposited in the last space. Sniffle's car was not there. "Great!" Nosemitt muttered; "what other homes could she have meant?" She thought of a couple and headed for the closer one, Evangelical Care– "the next best place before Heaven," as it was heavily advertised. There wasn't a prayer Sniffle would consider moving into a place like that one. The kitchen had been condemned twice; residents were not allowed to choose their own activities, let alone their own menus. Even independent types had to use wheelchairs when out of their rooms. The media had been on a campaign to shut the place down, but it was alive and nearby and Nosemitt checked out the parking lot. No familiar red car, thank goodness. She drove around the block to be sure, but she did not see Sniffle's car anywhere.

There weren't all that many residential facilities in Fondue or Sunford. In fact, there really was a great need for such places– but good ones, reasonably priced ones, caring ones, attentive ones, ones that were not in fact the next-to-the-last stop before Hell. Why was Sniffle contemplating looking into them? And then it occurred to Nosemitt: maybe she isn't scouting them out for herself. Maybe she got some bee in her bonnet about somebody else. That made far more sense, but why had she counted the paintings? Why was Nosemitt even asking herself these questions? "Really, you'd think I'd know better," she said to the steering wheel; and, as with almost all the objects Nosemitt addressed, this one agreed with her.

Sniffle's car was not anywhere near the shabby brick and frame converted motel that still had the old neon sign out front. It no longer worked, but once upon a time the place had been called SHADY ACRES. The name, though changed after a land re-zoning and sale of several acres to SHADY VALE, seemed appropriate. There was only one other Home that Nosemitt could think of within fifteen miles. She stopped for gasoline at one of the few remaining full service stations, had the tank filled, and drove past Sunford's city limits to Havencleft. There, indeed, was Sniffle's car, parked in the shade, near the door. "She hasn't lost all her faculties yet," Nosemitt said. The steering wheel did not respond, other than to cooperate in making the necessary turns.

Now Nosemitt faced another problem: should she go in? Would Sniffle be pleased or offended? Would they get into an argument and create a scene in front of a couple of muscular nurses? Would some burly attendant come running to put them both in padded cells? Such thoughts, brought on by having just seen a rerun of *Harvey*, made her sit in the car for several minutes. She watched through the tinted window as a frail old man with a walker inched his way out the door. He was dressed in brown checked pants and a green and red plaid shirt. A flowered tie hung well below his belt. Suddenly a large woman in an aide's uniform emerged and firmly collared the man, painstakingly forcing him back inside the building. Nosemitt regarded the scene as an omen and stayed put.

She studied the building itself. Pale buff brick on the front, it was dark brown aluminum siding the rest of the way around. The parking lot was large enough for about fifty cars and was swept clear of leaves and debris. Near the front entrance was a small patio and garden area with wrought iron tables and chairs, all unoccupied. A few late blooms, rust and yellow, drooped on the mums planted in a tiny circle around the patio. "It's not uncared for," Nosemitt thought out loud; "but why is she thinking about a Home already?"

A car pulled into the lot and a middle-aged couple got out, the woman carrying a suitcase and a handkerchief, the man looking grim and tired. *Someone died*, Nosemitt immediately realized and decided to stay in the car a while longer. *Their mother or father– hers, probably. They're coming to get her belongings, to settle things. What a depressing place to be.* She wondered how long Sniffle needed in order to realize she did not belong here yet. Maybe never. One could always hope for never.

She sat there for fifteen minutes, fifteen minutes that seemed like fifteen hours, watching an occasional leaf drift across the windshield, seeing an occasional delivery truck– milk, linens, produce– a thin parade of services, a trickle of life. No one seemed to come out, she noticed. People were absorbed into the place and never came out– except for the one old man who was too slow for his own good. She looked at her watch for the twentieth time and waited.

After forty-five minutes, she could stand it no more. She got out of the car slowly and she cautiously approached the front doors. She shaded her eyes, looked in through the dark glass of the doors, and finally opened one of them and went in. There was a small sign prohibiting smoking and a larger sign indicating the primary visiting hours. In very small letters was a message to indicate that in emergencies visiting hours might be extended or curtailed. In larger letters was a request for visitors to obtain passes from the receptionist. At the moment no such person was available. The receptionist's desk there in the foyer was bare except for a glass vase with an artificial rose, a telephone console, and a cup of pens and pencils. About ten feet away, separated from the desk by a gray and red area rug, was a cluster of black vinyl chairs and a walnut veneer table with half a dozen magazines. Nosemitt hesitated, looked down the three empty halls that converged here at the foyer, and went over to select a magazine. They were recent but Nosemitt had no interest in any of them. She walked casually down one hall, deserted and a little eerie. Why wasn't anyone around? All the doors along the hall were closed. The highly waxed floor echoed her own footsteps; the glary white walls reflected the glary fixtures overhead. The silence seemed unreal, silence more of a cemetery than of a home. Not a home, she corrected herself, a *Home* with a capital H. She went back to the waiting area and waited.

She was leafing absently through *Gerontological Newsbeat* when she became aware of a rustling coming near. She looked up and smiled at a nun in full habit sailing toward her, her hands busily plying her beads and her expression indicating that she was pleased to see Nosemitt. As the nun sat down beside her, Nosemitt smiled and said, "I didn't know this home was run by one of the orders." The sister smiled benevolently and patted Nosemitt's arm.

"May I ask which is your room?" the nun inquired.

"Oh, I don't live here," Nosemitt assured her.

"You are here to visit a dear one?"

"Well, not exactly," Nosemitt said, not knowing how to explain just what exactly she was doing there. "I'm waiting for a friend."

"Friends are a lovely thing, God wot," the nun assured her. "And which is her room?"

"She doesn't live here either. I am not sure whom she is visiting, but I am just waiting for her."

"How very sweet of you. You must be quite tired?"

"Not really," Nosemitt said, not seeing what would suggest that she was.

"May I see you to your room?" the nun asked politely, although it didn't seem entirely like a question.

Oh-oh, Nosemitt thought to herself; *she thinks I am crazy*. "I really think I'll wait right here," she said, trying to sound as pleasant and balanced and visitor-like as possible. There was a brisk no-nonsense sound of sensible shoes coming down the hall, and Nosemitt turned to see a tall nurse with a very red face.

"Sister, Sister, I've been looking for you. We need you in the dining room."

"Is there a problem, my dear?" Turning to Nosemitt, she said with only a hint of long-suffering, "Our work is never done. Bless you, and don't stay out here too long." She got up and left with the nurse.

"Don't stay out here too long? She still thinks I am supposed to be checked into a room. Where is Sniffle?" Nosemitt got up and walked slowly down one of the other halls. There seemed to be a few offices along this corridor, although no one was visible in any of them. After about forty or fifty feet, the hall intersected with another, the new one apparently being the start of the residents' rooms. Nosemitt wandered very slowly past the open doors, embarrassed to look in but unable to keep from doing so. In one room a young woman was gently brushing the long white hair of one of the residents. Despite the tenderness with which she brushed, the scene was grim and lonely. From another room came the incessant soft moaning of pain, muted by unbearable fatigue. A tattered and grimy pink robe lay on the floor of that room. Nosemitt wondered if she should go in and pick it up. Something told her not to.

In another room a small balding lady rocked and rocked on her bed, cradling an imaginary infant. She cooed and crooned to the invisible child and clucked and smiled at the inaudible response. Nosemitt was moved to tears and was worried that she might disturb the woman. She moved on. She passed by two rooms with sleeping inmates– she hoped they were merely asleep; and at the end of this hall, in the room on the right, she saw again the middle-aged couple. They were packing the contents of a few dresser drawers and one closet, all that remained of a once full life– she hoped it had been a full life. Then she came to another intersection and turned left.

step four: taking leave of salt, welcoming drying

There was the dining room. Nosemitt worried for a moment that the nun would see her and order her confined to a room, but then she saw Sniffle standing and talking with a young woman in a bright blue well-tailored suit. Judging from their expressions and the occasional bursts of laughter, they seemed to be having a pleasant conversation. Sniffle happened to turn around and was very surprised to see Nosemitt. She waved excitedly for her to join them, and Nosemitt breathed a sigh of relief.

"I didn't expect to see you here!" Sniffle said, but obviously she was pleased.

"I might say the same," Nosemitt replied, smiling at the young administrator, who was reaching out to shake hands, ready to introduce herself.

"This is Corinne Webster," Sniffle said to Nosemitt; "she is in charge of programming and public relations for a number of residential centers."

"Oh," Nosemitt said, unable to figure out what was going on exactly.

"We're quite pleased that Ms Sniffle has agreed to exhibit her paintings here. We're always looking for ways to stimulate the residents' minds and also to have some variety here in the dining hall. We think we can easily accommodate twenty or thirty paintings."

"You came here to scout out the *walls*?" Nosemitt asked.

"Yes," Sniffle said, pleased at the space. Nosemitt did not know whether to laugh or be angry; she looked frustrated.

"Oh," Sniffle said, realizing. "I did it again, didn't I? Just left you puzzling." Nosemitt nodded. Corinne looked puzzled too.

"All she said to me," Nosemitt explained to the program director, "was that she was going to scout out the Home. Perhaps you are too young to know what that suggests to me."

"You thought she was checking in here?" Corinne asked, chuckling. "No, I understand. My mother thinks I'm going to commit her every time she forgets anything. All of her friends half joke about my getting them group rates. I know what you thought."

"I clearly counted the paintings first," Sniffle said mildly defensively, as if that explained anything. "Anyway, the space and light here are just fine. I'll be glad to come hang the work next week."

"We do have insurance but we rarely have any damage," Corinne said; "but if a resident should happen to break some glass or dent a frame, we will replace whatever or we will buy the painting."

"That's fairer than a good many galleries," Sniffle said, pleased.

A rustling sound announced the arrival of the sister. Corinne smiled at her and said, "Not yet, Sister Eustachia, but we'll be done soon." The nun turned and went to one of the dining tables, sat down and pulled out a testament from her sleeve, and began to read.

"Will there be a test on this?" she asked Corinne.

"No, Sister, no test. You read the next chapter and we'll have a little talk soon."

"She is a resident here?" Nosemitt asked, appalled. "She isn't part of the administration?"

"Sister Eustachia is not even Catholic," Corinne confided. "She decided a few months ago that she was called to be a nun. We had to rent a habit for her from one of the costume shops, and she insists that I am her teacher."

"How did she come by her name?" Nosemitt asked.

"It's a long story," Corinne evaded; "let's just say she enjoys medical books. It could have been much worse."

Another resident came into the dining room and sat down with Sister Eustachia. The two of them pored over the verses together and the newcomer toyed with the rosary, wrapping it in bracelet fashion around her wrist. "We have a new novice," Sister Eustachia declared. "We must have her join our study."

"Oh, yes," sighed the novice-to-be. Corinne looked moderately horrified. She had hoped the course of study was nearing an end.

"She will be Sister Epidermis," Eustachia pronounced, "and she will be my assistant." The future Sister Epidermis was thrilled. She turned her face away to keep the moment to herself and, in turning, caught sight of some peeling paint on one of the support columns in the middle of the dining room. She slid over to a chair by the column and, pretending that she was just sitting there quietly, began surreptitiously to pull off little strips and larger sections of paint, dropping them onto the floor,

"Does she think she can't be seen?" Sniffle whispered.

"We find little piles of paint strips all around the place. We always know she was there. It's just one of her little peculiarities."

"You must give up paint peeling for Lent this year," Sister Eustachia loudly announced to her new assistant. "It will be your sacrifice." Epidermis almost burst into tears and was not sure she wished to be a sister after all.

"Now, now, my dear," Eustachia said, hurrying over to her, "you know that Lent does not last forever. Think with what renewed vigor you can return to this work after a short abstinence. You will be so happy, and God and Corinne will be pleased too." Epidermis did not know how long Lent lasted and so was not entirely convinced.

"Besides, we shall be so cheerfully occupied studying our testaments and our prayer books and you especially will love the hymnals. You shall teach me to sing." Epidermis began immediately to sing *A Hundred Bottles Of Beer On the Wall.*

"The entire cloister will be one of great interest some day," Sniffle suggested. Corinne, potential mother superior, looked more pained than ever.

"I thought she was in charge here," Nosemitt said, still recalling her fears of being forcibly inserted into a room. "I felt certain she had sized me up as a sure thing for the padded walls. I feel rather badly about seeing her like this; she seems so real as a nun."

"She is more real as a nun than as anything else so far," Corinne said. "This is the first time she has taken a positive interest in others since she has been here. We regard it as a relatively good thing."

"Than anything else so far?" Sniffle repeated. "What else has she been?"

"For a very short time she thought she was a clock. She decided that ticking was the only way she would communicate,except for twice a day when she crowed. She said that crowing was a more natural alarm than a gong or chime or buzz. She woke everyone at dawn and then crowed again at sunset."

"And how did that end?" Nosemitt asked, somewhat alarmed herself.

"A very hostile resident here suggested that clocks could get their hands broken. She converted immediately."

"From clock to Catholic?" Sniffle asked.

"Oh no, from clock to file cabinet."

"You're not serious!" Nosemitt insisted.

"I wish!" said Corinne. "She definitely proclaimed herself a file cabinet and walked up and down the halls carrying empty folders. Someone told her that file cabinets remain in place in one room. She stayed in her room for two days and came out, announcing that she was on casters. The same hostile resident took care of this incarnation too. He told her he would personally donate all office equipment to the State Mental Hospital. Many of our residents have known that place directly or indirectly and it is a potent threat."

"At least he still has his wits," Sniffle said admiringly.

"That's terrible," Nosemitt said. "There is some grim humor in all this, but it is terribly serious and sad. Isn't there any way to help her without physical and mental threats?"

"We see our role in her life as providers of a safe environment for her remaining days. We can't prevent residents from saying all kinds of things to each other, but we would not let her get attacked in any physical sense. We kept trying to find a human personality she would enjoy– without success– until she decided herself that she was called to be a nun. As I said, it has been the most positive thing she has done since she arrived here. But I see I had better discuss whatever she has settled on today. She is starting to get frantic at my being occupied. Thanks again, Ms. Sniffle, and I'll see you next week."

They looked over to see Sister Eustachia in tears, chewing one bead of her rosary, indifferent to Epidermis's efforts to console her; and they saw her brighten immediately as Corinne sat down beside her. Tears vanished, the dent in the rosary bead was blessed, and the three women began to read together. "And what is meant by tidings of great joy, do you think?" Corinne was asking as Nosemitt and Sniffle walked toward the doors.

"That we are going to have a new order," Eustachia beamed, "and we will save Sister Epidermis."

step five: smoking

Epidermis pulled a pack of illegal cigarettes from her pocket and lit one, throwing it immediately on the floor. "I wouldn't count on having that show next week," Nosemitt whispered to Sniffle as they headed together down the silent halls.

~ Miss Billie Dances

It helps if one can approach nursing homes and their residents with at least a shred of a sense of humor. With all the pathos housed in those rooms, if humor can be found, it helps to laugh at it. There are memorable citizens of many worlds living together in disconnected and often discordant little segments of the long days. Everyone needs to find a friend.

I thought I had been found as one myself one day. I had often seen Miss Billie walking herself along in her wheelchair. Many residents get around faster rolling their chairs with their feet than with their arms, and she and Mom are two such persons. Miss Billie seemed particularly unhappy one afternoon; and as I passed her in the hall on the way to see Mom, she stopped me with such pathetic words that I could not pass her by. "Please, won't you stop and talk with me? I am so lonely, and no one is visiting me today." I had seen her son with her a few times, but he was not there then; I knew she missed him.

She asked me whom I was there to visit, and I told her. She acknowledged knowing my mother, but then she said, "It is so hard for me to be here. I am so angry with my family for putting me here when they know I still could manage for myself." Yes, it was very sad, I agreed.

"I still can cook," she said, "but I probably don't clean as well as I used to. I don't need to be here just because I can't keep up with the housework. It would cost a whole lot less just to hire someone to come in and clean. And of course I miss dancing. I was quite a dancer in my younger days. I really do miss that. Here I just sit in this wheelchair all day. I get no exercise. And I miss reading. My eyes aren't quite what they were."

I asked her what kind of dancing she liked best, and she told me that she liked all kinds but especially ballet. Her eyes lit up as she recalled some of the ballet costumes she had worn in her dancing days. "A long time ago, now," she sighed; "but my memory is excellent and I remember it all. They need to let me go home."

She asked my name, and I told her. "And whom are you here to see?" she asked. I told her again. "Oh, yes, I know your mother. Whom are you here to see?" "My mother," I said, smiling.

"You haven't told me your name," she said. I told her. "I'll bet you'd never guess that I was once a dancer." I assured her that I would not have guessed it. It was hard not to grin.

"Well, whatever your name is, please visit with me again. I have an excellent memory for names and faces. Whom are you here to see?" I chuckled all the way to Mom's room. If not, I'd have been crying.

~ Miss Billie Talks With God

Miss Billie was a woman of moods and of temper. Often enough one could find her in the hall in front of her bedroom door telling God just what she thought of the plan. "O, my Lord God, thou hast allowed us to live but hast not taught us how to die. I am ready, God, but you will not have me. Show me how to die, I beg of you. Please, God, teach me how to die. I am an old woman, and no one wants me down here. No one visits me. No one helps me."

As I passed by, she once again called out to me to help her. I was leery, but I stopped to ask her how I could help her. "Are you stupid?" she demanded. It was a surprising response.

"No, I don't think so," I said; "but I can't help you if I don't know what you need."

"You ARE stupid," she said. "You are the stupidest stupid person I have ever met."

I have heard enough of that from my mother; this woman was not going to start in on me, too. "I am going to ask you what you need one more time and then I am leaving. If you don't want to tell me what you need, that is fine."

"You are an idiot!" she said. "Of course you know what I need. Even a stupid idiot like you can figure it out."

"Well, then," I said, "you shouldn't ask an idiot. As far as I'm concerned, you should go on asking God to help you. Have a nice day."

"Wait a moment, young lady. Just one minute."

"Yes?"

"I asked for your help."

"Yes, you did. In a rather odd way, but you did ask. I don't work here; I am visiting my mother, and you want me to help you but won't say how. I don't even know if you want something I am allowed to do."

"It's easy. Even an idiot can do it."

"What is it?"

"Connect my oxygen tank, you fool! I can hardly talk!"

So I had noticed.

~ Hard-Driving Miss Billie

Elderly people, like every other category of human being, come in all flavors– bland, sweet, salty, peppery, buttery– and in all textures. They can be smooth or rough, biting or gentle; they can be all of the above within a given five minutes. The main difference I see between the elderly flavors and the younger ones is that many inhibitions have disappeared by later life. Coherent thoughts that form come screaming out at any nearby living thing, as gentle observations do in sweeter tones. For that matter, incoherent thoughts come out in the same mix of ways.

Miss Billie one fine afternoon was in the mood again for a little conversation, fortunately not with me. She pedaled her wheel chair across the corridor to challenge Miss Bobbie to a conversation. Now, Miss Billie was well known throughout her wing for her caustic style. No one ever wanted to converse with her, least of all Miss Bobbie. The latter said quite firmly, "No."

"I said I wanted to have a conversation with you," Miss Billie repeated. "Are you deaf?"

"And I said No, you old bat," Miss Bobbie replied. She too was well known for not mincing words.

Miss Billie stared long and hard at her opponent. She wheeled forward for an in-your-face repetition of her offer. "I do want to talk," she shouted.

"Go talk to yourself," Leon shrieked. "Leave us all alone."

"I wasn't speaking to you, you fool," Miss Billie spat over her shoulder. She rolled backward and then pedaled furiously forward right into Miss Bobbie again, her head thrust forward like a charmless cobra springing out of its basket. "Talk with me," she ordered.

Feeling confident, thanks to Leon, Miss Bobbie told her to get the hell out of her sight. Mistake.

Deeply offended by profanity not her own, Miss Billie looked shocked for a moment, blinked a few times, and made her decision. "You are dead," she shouted. "You are dead and too stupid to know it. What an absurd fool you are, thinking you are alive. I see you but not for long. You are dead and about to be buried."

Miss Bobbie burst into tears. "Damn you," she screamed. "Get away from me. I hate you; I hate you. You are evil!" Miss Billie laughed and pedaled away, announcing that Miss Bobbie was dead.

That episode occurred a year ago, and now Miss Bobbie can relax. Miss Billie finally found acceptance from God, and presumably there is an angel somewhere willing to have a conversation with her. Maybe an imp.

~ Sephia

Mom's first roommate was a soft-spoken but husky-voiced woman from Greece. She was always pleasant and patient, but she talked only now and then. Not only was she Mom's roommate; she also was a tablemate at all meals. In that first year, my mother still attempted conversation with a few, but Sephia was not one of them, much to the confusion and disappointment of that gentle woman. Part of the problem, if not all of it, seemed to be that if any of us spoke with Sephia, Mom would get openly jealous. "You here for me," she would say all too clearly, "not that one." Sephia would smile and shrug.

One of the long-running issues between my mother and me was my haircut. You would think she would give up on trying to make me look like her after a few years at the longest; but she never stopped urging me get rid of my short straight home-cut "style" (if one can call it that). She offered to "give it shape," curl it, pay for a professional cut, anything, everything; but I stuck with my father's principle of the natural look. I did not consider haircuts anything other than natural, as in my paternal family line there are several barbers. Frequent haircuts were totally normal and natural. End of issue, as far as I was and am concerned. You may think this is irrelevant, but it isn't.

One evening, while residents were sitting at the dining room tables waiting for dinner to be served, Mom started in about my hair. "Cut," she said. "Bad," she said. She shook her head as if to ask when would I ever realize how important looks are. It was then that I learned what Sephia's voice sounded like, how deep and relaxing it was. How pleasant. She leaned forward and stroked my hair, smiled warmly, and said like an ancient Melina Mercouri with laryngitis, "I luff your hair!"

Mom glared at us both, but Sephia made my day.

~ Mr. Parks

Mom liked Mr. Parks. He was very much the gentleman, always neatly dressed and courteous to everyone. He always smiled. He was highly educated, something my mother oddly fantasized that she was too, having gone to secretarial school for several months back when she had just graduated from high school. In fact, going to secretarial school did move her to being the most highly educated member of her family; but it did not overly impress others.

Quite frequently Mr. Parks would wheel himself into the dining room where Mom and I would be playing a game of dominos or cards, and she would always smile and wave at him. He unfailingly smiled and wheeled straight to the television set. If he had a visitor, which he often did, you could hear rational discussion going on and you might well wonder why he was installed in the nursing home. He did not lack for caring family or apparent ability. Actually, he didn't really need the wheelchair; he was quite able to take himself for walks around the halls.

It was only when he had no company that you saw another side of Mr. Parks. His calm intelligence seemed to melt away; he became instantly confused and would wander into others' rooms, unable to find his own. His clear eyes would go blank, and his words would become repetitive and meaningless. He might ask over and over for his wife or for his meal, his wife having just left after having lunch with him. Then you could understand that this was a man who could not cope on his own, could not do much with any degree of success or safety. In the comfort of family presence, he was renewed.

He is another of the tragic victims of dementia, a once highly competent and successful human being reduced now to a fraction of himself. What was good in his case, though, bothered me with respect to its implications. Because he had been a well known member of the community, he was treated with uniform kindness by all. One never saw him being handled roughly; one never heard him being told to shut up; one never saw a speck of unkindness or disrespect.

That is how it should be for every person there, but that is not how it is for most. We need not little aristocracies based on station in life but democracies of a high order, where everyone is valued and truly cared for.

Too often as I am leaving after visiting my mother, I hear one aide or another belittling a cringing resident or a blankly staring one. Whether or not that old woman in the bed understands what is being said to her, she needs to be held in respect. Yes, she is a burden; but she is a human one who did not ask to be in the condition she now finds herself. She is the equal of Mr. Parks and of us all.

~ Mistaken Identity

There are many reasons that I hate nursing homes, most of them having to do with the treatment of residents and the differences between public appearance and private reality. I also have a personal grudge. First a bit of background: My mother is thirty years older than I am. For her entire life she has looked years younger than her actual age; and we all have been pleased for her, since being mistaken for a woman of sixty when she was eighty made her elated. In her nineties, she looks on good days perhaps a decade younger; and when she dresses up for a party, she looks even younger, though not anywhere near as young as she did. On most days now, she certainly looks more than eighty or eighty-five. Having taken care of her for three stressful years, I also no longer look as young as I did prior to her stroke; but I do not look as if I am a hundred and twenty-five. Yet because she called me mother, countless aides and social workers at the nursing home would say to me, "So this is your daughter?" There I was, wheeling my ninety-year old "daughter" around the halls, leaving with car keys in hand after a visit, known to have a full-time job; and they are asking me with a straight face if she is my child. To say I was offended is not even the top of the tip of any iceberg.

Worse yet, the same social worker asked me on two different occasions if she could help me to my own room!

Worst of all, several aides thought that both my sister and my sister-in-law were my daughters. Well, maybe not worst of all. I think the first took the prize, that anyone would think I was my very own grandmother. My sense of humor shut down completely and I was extremely indignant. Fortunately a few of the nurses whispered to me, "We have some real idiots on the staff." I agreed with them, but the subject remained a sore spot. After the first couple of times, I found myself saying that yes, I was her mother and that I was indeed one hundred and twenty-five but in great shape thanks to a diet of dark chocolate and caffeine-free soda. Then they probably really wanted to escort me somewhere– somewhere out of the way and with soft walls.

One young aide asked me why Mom would call me mother if I was her daughter. She must have been on her first day of the job if she did not understand what dementia can come up with. "She had a stroke," I would say to her; "she doesn't always say what she means." I would just get blank looks.

These are the people whose observational skills can be of such great importance in helping their charges, mostly frail elderly people who can be difficult to understand. If they can look at me and think that I am in my hundreds and scampering around the building wheeling this youngster of ninety, how in the world can anyone trust any of their observations about anything? I have no answer to this question.

~ A Failed Motive

Yet another in my list of reasons for taking on the role of caregiver was what I once hoped would be role modeling for my adult children. I believed very strongly in the principle of family care and felt a need to live up to my values. Not only did I not want anyone I knew to be placed in institutional care, I did not want to think of it for my own future self either. I didn't see how I could expect to be cared for in a time of need unless I was willing to provide the same. I wanted to be a good role model. Well, let's not pretend that life necessarily works that way.

It took very little time in the caregiver capacity for me to know that even though my relationship with my children is not the same as my relationship with my own parents, I never would want them to have the deeply ambivalent feelings for me that I have had for Mom. For all that I too can say now that I don't want to be a burden to anyone, I have no idea of how I will feel when in fact I cannot take care of myself. I am afraid of what I might become. Will I be a shrew? a self-made martyr? a body alive only in the strictest and narrowest meaning of the word? Might I be pleasant and appreciative? easy to deal with? loving and cooperative? Quite honestly, none of us can know how we will be when our known self shatters.

We clearly have dementia running rampant in our genes, and yet we have our shining stars who light a different possibility. I am not a gambler. I don't trust the odds to work in my favor. At the same time, I truly detest the care system that currently prevails in our society. It works well for some who are totally dependent and mentally absent; they sleep away their final days or years apparently unaware of the level of care they are receiving. It also can work well for those who retain their faculties and their ability to communicate intelligently. They can elect a nursing home, speak meaningfully, and make their complaints and satisfactions known. It is the large number in the middle, those who have lost some or all of their competence to speak for themselves and who yet remain aware of all that is happening around and to them, who are the source of my personal fears and anxieties.

I have watched too many nurses and aides, unaware of my presence, as they treat some wide-eyed gibberish-speaking old woman with laughter, contempt, harshness. When they become aware of my presence, instant change! The tone of voice becomes soothing; the language is loving; the body touches are gentle. Do they have so little respect for themselves as human beings and so little awareness of the meaning of their behavior that they think they fool us onlookers?

That is when I feel guilty about having my mother in any institution and why I do understand her outbursts, *"Take me home!"* I know that I will feel the same way if I am ever in such a place, surrounded by such behavior and attitude. I will be angry if my children ignore me. I fear that I will resent how little time they will find for me.

If it is enough now that we spend a few days a year together, living as two of them do more than two thousand miles away, how could I expect them to change? Their daily lives do not include me now; why would their days include me then? It is a coldly frightening prospect. I would not want all the burden of my own future to fall on just one of my children, the one who lives closest. I don't want any of them to resent me or to be disgusted at whatever changes come about. I believe that love can overcome such feelings. I am prepared, but not really prepared, to be disappointed in my probable failure as a role model.

I'd like to think that friends can plan an old age together. Many of us talk about just such a thing– purchasing an apartment building and hiring someone to manage it and oversee the lot of us in our separate accommodations. But will we ever do such a thing? I doubt that our need and timing will coincide. I am afraid it is just talk. For those of us who live alone, it needs to be more than talk.

It is a problem filled with reality but it seems to have only fantasy solutions right now. Yes, we want to plan for the future; and yes, we want in this moment not to become inevitable burdens. In all likelihood, our good intentions will fail unless we plan solidly and build concretely. Perhaps they will fail anyway, life being the unpredictable matter that it is. The role modeling we do now has little to do with the future. Our children's lives are as different from ours as ours were different from those of our grandparents. It is possible that my generation will prove to be the last to have a significant number of individuals who accept the role modeling of our predecessors, willing to sacrifice personal freedom for the sake of another, although I am sure there will always be exceptions.

The chief hope right now seems to lie in the direction of research into what constitutes a healthy living environment for the elderly and needy. The flaw will be in the reality of what quality of person will be drawn to work in such an environment. Ambiance means little when loving care is missing. I think about what my mother most values now: time and love, not material gifts. She smiles and says thank you to anyone who presents her with anything, but the only objects she really cherishes are the little stuffed animals and dolls she can hold close and talk to, pretending that they are her beloved. She always did love toys and dolls; there is no change in this respect, except that she values them even more. I am not a doll person; if I try to predict what might bring me comparable comfort, I suppose I hope I will be surrounded by my favorite paintings and able still to read and speak. Mostly I hope to retain my mind and remain independent. If not, then I hope for a quick and painless end. I think that will be the best role modeling I can do.

~ Caveats

I believe I know the value of my experiences with my mother. Stressful as they were, and as much as I might often have wished that they could have been more pleasant all of the time, the fact is that I do not regret the three years. However, if anyone were to ask me for advice– and not many will ever want it– I would ask them first of all, Are you willing to hear the down sides before we get to the positives? Get acquainted with both realities, and then allow for personal variations. Only you know what you can handle, but at least get an idea of what that might be.

I would start with this one: do not count on family help. You may get it; you may be blessed with a wonderfully cooperative batch of relatives who believe in sharing the work. Just don't count on it. Of course they will have other obligations, and that is natural and right; but be prepared for them to put even their minor recreational needs first. Expect that coming in to give you relief will not be among their top priorities. If you can accept that as a realistic possibility, you have a greater chance to avoid later bitterness; and if you are among the lucky, it will turn out to be a false warning. Just don't stop asking them to help, unless doing so does you in.

Remind yourself frequently that your sanity matters every bit as much as that of the person for whom you are caring. Don't let anyone make you feel guilty about getting away for regular breaks. If, like me, you aren't happy about having strangers come into your home for more than a few hours, let alone a few days, look into the availability in nearby facilities for short-term stays. Many places offer this welcome opportunity to caregivers; ask about respite care. When my youngest son got married, Mom had a reservation for ten days'accommodation; and I had one of my rare breaks of more than two or three hours. The beach was never so welcome as it was then, never more beautiful.

Do not let others prevent you from speaking the truth. Some will be willing to hear you out, but many will not. They would prefer to think that you are a natural at caregiving and that that is why you are doing it. They will be eager to let you feel that you are doing a great job– and you probably are– but they don't want to know the details. Tell some of them anyway, especially family. You can spare your friends all you want, but they are more likely to be willing to listen and offer support. If your care recipient can understand you, allow him or her to know when things get too demanding. You have rights, too.

Be prepared for many people to assure you that they know exactly what you are going through. Many of them really do. Having been immersed in three different levels of caregiving, though, I can tell you that there is a huge difference between around the clock care and taking a shift every day, just as there is an equally large gulf between regular shifts and daily visits, let alone irregular visits. All levels of care will become difficult and stressful in their own ways, but very few people who haven't taken on exactly what you have taken on really do know what is involved. Don't forget, too, that the quality of the relationship before the illness makes a major difference, as does the ability level of both parties to handle the imaginable and the unimaginable things that come along.

Find things to do just for yourself. All of my painting and all the art shows went on hold when Mom moved in. Paint fumes were too toxic to risk exposing her to them. I did wood carving instead, and I would work on the porch where she could see me but not keep asking me the time. (By the way, I had put a clock where she could see it easily, but she refused to remember that it was there.)

Do not expect that your furniture or carpeting will ever get clean again. Maybe you will find that only one room gets abused, and maybe you even know how to restore everything. Nowhere that Mom wheeled herself in the house was exempt from marks, only some of which disappeared. This may be more a reflection on me than on her. I am not devoted to cleaning and restoring, even when the money might be available.

If you are the full-time caregiver and are independently wealthy, money may not be an issue for you. I had been living the stereotyped struggling artist's life and could not have afforded to take Mom in and stop working without her contributing to household expenses. Don't be afraid to cover that topic with any others in your family who have a voice in the relevant financial decisions. If you are keeping someone from a nursing institution, you are saving that person and the family many tens of thousands of dollars every year; and that is at current prices.

Make use of technology! Whether it is the telephone, the computer, or whatever might be the big new item, if it helps you survive the daily eroding of your life and mind, try it. And read. Work puzzles. Do what you can to keep yourself mentally healthy. Perhaps I should add, Buy art! Enhance your visual outlook. Write. Play. Yes, make sure you play. Dream. Think about those dreams, and don't take every one literally. Find their virtues and use them to help you through the difficult times. Expect many.

Take advantage of the opportunity to get to know yourself and your new live-in companion. Know why you are doing what you have offered to do or been manipulated into doing. Let's hope it is the former.

If a support group appeals to you, join one. If counseling might help to relieve the stress, go.

Finally, don't be afraid to decide to stop. You alone know your own limits. You make the decision, but pay attention to your own body's signals and your own mind's cues. Your life matters, even when some people might prefer to think otherwise. I'd like to repeat that: *your life matters.*

~ Got a Life?

Let's just state at the outset that I know I am a judgmental person. I don't even apologize for it; I believe we were given minds that make distinctions and evaluations for our own self-preservation. We can't make intelligent choices without declaring some things better than others, some life paths more suitable and appealing, some people healthier for us to befriend, and some acts better or worse according to our own code of values. There is nothing wrong with evaluating. Listening to the evaluations of others and heeding their various, not to mention contradictory, orders as the main method we have of deciding our own course of actions is entirely different. Don't do it! (You can ignore me, of course, if you wish.)

As an exhibiting artist for over twenty years, I heard about as wide a spectrum of response and advice as I can imagine exists. My work has been called everything from powerful to challenging to a depressingly large number of four-letter words, none complimentary. I have been thanked countless times for expressing what others have felt but not visualized, and I have been accused of perpetrating a fraud upon art judges and the art-buying public. I have been urged and encouraged to keep on, and I have been equally urged to give it all up and get a life. The only technique for emotional survival if one is at all sensitive is to fortify oneself and learn to dismiss all responses as each individual's personal projective. What they say speaks far more to their needs and fears and understandings than it ever does to the intent or quality of the work. The acclaim is briefly pleasing; indifference is meaningless; the insults are briefly aggravating. Objective truth lies nowhere.

It's when the praise and the attacks switch from the work to the person that the real line has to be drawn, firmly drawn. An artist is not evil because some viewers see evil in the images. An artist is not great simply because the painting of the barn against the sunset looks So Real. For some people, art has to depict physical reality; for others it depicts emotional reality; for others, intellectual exercise. For some, it is a spiritual journey. Viewers have every right to their personal preferences, but they need to put their reactions in perspective and figure out what they are saying about themselves. When the projective becomes all that matters, it has nothing to do with the artist.

To all those people, family or friends or total strangers, who urged me to get a real life, I simply have had to learn to turn my back and continue on my way. Our lives are not the same; but, believe me, I have a real life, and so do you.

It is the same everywhere, not just in the art world. Many teachers complain bitterly that they have no "real" life; their days and nights are spent directly or indirectly on school matters. They want to define their real lives by what they do when they are not working, but work is at least a third of their day. Better to redefine what you mean by *real* than to dismiss so much of your life as not real. People outside the current educational milieu rarely understand how demanding and strenuous the day of a teacher is; they don't understand that frequent holidays and the other days off for kids when staff goes on working can only begin to relieve the stress. Teachers, on the other hand, too often have warped (read *completely erroneous*) ideas of how difficult the days and nights of other professionals are, much less those of people living less conventional lives altogether. They seem to think that everyone else is earning a fortune for doing practically nothing. Such thinking has little to do with reality and everything to do with feeling deprived of some essential quality in their own lives– usually in their cases, solid blocks of undemanding time.

As a caregiver, I have run up against the same kinds and range of reactions, positive and negative, that exist everywhere else– with one difference. Caregivers draw a level of emotional response far deeper than what I had ever encountered before. People tend to think that you are either a saint or a martyr, and they don't approve of martyrs. Those who think you are a saint tend to be the ones who, faced with the same challenge, would want to say Yes, whether they actually could and did so or not. Perhaps they have tried it and found themselves unable to continue. They approve of the implicit code of ethical behavior and they assume your motives are theirs. They empathize from their own frame of reference, and sometimes they are right but not always.

It's the crowd of antagonistic people who amaze me. Whether it was my mother's friends telling me that Mom did not deserve such care, peers telling me to call it quits, strangers challenging my competence, other strangers demanding to know why my need to be a martyr, individuals ordering me to *get a life*, or just out and out hostility– all of these reactions and more deserve only one reply: why does it matter to you? Seriously, Why? What is threatening you?

I am neither saint nor martyr. I have plenty of human emotion about what Mom and I went through together. I have no illusion that it was forced upon me and that I am simply the patient bearer of the burden she became. I took her on voluntarily, and I don't hesitate to label it a sacrifice. I have had some criticism even for using that word, as if it proves my martyrdom. It does not. I would ask, did ask, the person who said that the word showed that I just wanted to be a martyr, *Define sacrifice.* Her answer was that sacrifice is a needless destruction of one's own life in a spurious search for martyrdom. How convenient a definition and, really, I can't help thinking how shallow a one it is! But it is a personal projective, nothing more.

To my thinking, sacrifice means a willing giving up of something for a greater good. That greater good, in my situation, was experience and insight and the hope of a loving relationship before the end. You are free to think otherwise, but I believe that those valuable pursuits are among the many things that real life is all about.

~ Items for Someone's Notebook

I spent a lot of time observing, fascinated by my mother's language abilities and disabilities. There were some patterns but more apparent randomnesses in what she could or would say, but there was little doubt about what she could or would hear. Mom had been gradually losing some of her hearing prior to her stroke, but she had responsibly taken herself to an ear specialist and willingly used hearing aids. Not the least of her reasons was that she disapproved of the fact that both of her sisters avoided using theirs, and she wanted to be the good girl. She held onto the illusion that they admired her for it, never recognizing their irritation with her. I would love for them to know that after their deaths, she threw one of her two hearing aids away and lost the other.

Mild deafness in a stubborn elderly person is a definite advantage. If I was talking on the phone a room away, she could hear me. If I spoke within two feet of her to tell her that I was going to be on the phone for a few minutes, she would look blank, shrug her shoulders, and assure me that she had no idea of what I had just said and would not let me move until she could hear. We cut that game short very quickly.

At her doctor appointments she beamed when he softly told her how well she was doing and claimed profound deafness when he tried to encourage her to accept sitters and let me get out more often. Again, Mom was never subtle, and her hearing quality has been of less interest to me than her speech issues.

Why does she remember and say no names but her own? Is it pure self-centeredness of the unpleasant kind, or is there literally a special place in the brain for *ME*? She can name her significant dates— or is that one of her numbers things? She knows who we all are but almost never knows our names. If I show her a list of names, she always correctly matches them to photos. Why can she sometimes say nothing coherent or recognizable and other times speak an entire paragraph as she would have before the stroke? Every year at her birthday party, she gives a loving thank you speech that brings tears to our eyes. Again, excitement brings back some of her former ability. Who is looking into that? How common is it among the stroke victim population?

One afternoon, back in the hospital intensive care unit for another of her hemorrhages, she suddenly launched into an hour of incredibly clear conversation. At one point she addressed the nurse who had come into the room. "Excuse me, please, but is there a commode in here? I don't think I can walk to the bathroom." The nurse and I were both astonished, but her language continued at that quality and then abruptly faded. I tried to find out if she had been put on some new medication while there, but no one seemed aware of any. (Do not ever count on records. They are frequently wrong, often lacking essential details, and depressingly often allegedly not ever written, despite requirements. See "Off the Record".)

What besides random reconnections explains the phenomenon of her short-term reawakening? Why are we assuming that it always IS random? She had hemorrhaged and had had blood transfusions; did the new blood play a part, if only for an hour? What bothers me is that my questions were treated with derision. Who is willing to see if there are connections that medicine has yet to find? Who will listen to the questions of ordinary citizens thrust into caregiver roles who notice all kinds of things, large and small, and want to understand? Why pencil? Why Humphrey? Researchers, where you?

~ Off the Record

If there is one phrase that drives me crazy, whether it comes from institutions like hospitals and nursing homes and banks or from individuals like doctors and tellers and managers, it is this: *It isn't in the records.* I want to scream, "WHY NOT?" and I am not a screamer. It takes a whole lot of frustration before it ever occurs to me to want to scream or shout, and even then I don't do it. I am inclined to express my anger softly. I could wish for a bit more appreciation for this quality.

WHY? I want to know does every staff member you encounter upon entering any medical facility want you to sit down and give them endless bits of information and then apparently scrap them all? WHY, even before we produced any records to keep, did my mother have to wait six hours in the emergency room before being seen when it was already almost certain that she had had a stroke and it was already known that immediate treatment could prevent some of the damage? That is really a separate question, but it too inspires screaming, and it brings us to the records again.

Even a few days after Mom was finally admitted to a room, half the nurses attending her did not know she had had a stroke. "Oh?" they said. "It isn't in her records."

Stray doctors would wander into her room and begin questioning her, then look at me when they couldn't understand her answers. "Stroke," I would say. "Oh?" they said. "It isn't in her records." Scream! Why had they even come in? What WAS in the records beside her name?

When she fell and cracked three vertebrae, she needed fusion surgery. The doctor's orders were that she not be gotten out of bed for several days. On day two, I arrived to find her being walked down the hall. "She isn't supposed to be out of bed," I said, puzzled and worried. "Oh?" they said. "It isn't in her records." The surgeon was very angry, and so was I.

Day one in the rehab unit after that surgery, the charge nurse said to me, "Well, she won't need to be here long. Be glad it wasn't serious." It was surgery for a broken neck; I thought that was serious. "Oh?" she said. "It isn't in her records." I hope that by now you are screaming softly or loudly with me.

When we checked her out of the rehab unit of the nursing home, I had to participate in an exit interview; and I had a number of specific complaints to register– three single-spaced typed pages, to be exact. The team as a group got very hostile to some of my remarks and said, "You are complaining about us, but you have never told us why she was here in the first place. You were supposed to give us detailed information, but nothing is in her records." GO BEYOND MERE SCREAMING.

I had answered every one of their questions, filled out every one of their dozens of forms, as had her doctors, and they were blaming me for their having nothing in their records? It is preposterous and well worth screaming about, but I quietly told them what I thought of them and their nursing home. I sent my three pages to the Director, who never directly acknowledged receiving them. However, the medical director, whom I did hold in high respect, wrote to thank me for bringing all of the problems to their attention and said it would be the topic of staff meetings. Whether anyone took it seriously is another matter. I doubt it.

I took Mom for a follow-up appointment with her doctor and told him of my experience. He looked confused and pulled out his copy of her records as faxed to him by both the hospital and the nursing home. Every detail was there. Every item specifically recorded. The reasons for her surgery and the kind of surgery required. The medical orders for how long she needed to be confined to bed. The pain medication she was to have and how frequently. (I had had to fight them to get her the prescribed meds when she first arrived and was in intense pain. They brought it two hours later, even though the medical director himself had ordered them to bring it immediately.)

So the issue isn't whether or not they have records. Clearly they do. The information does not go poof in the night, nor does it vanish into Faxland never to emerge again. Perhaps the problem is more often that the immediate care providers don't read. They don't even look. They would rather say, "Oh? It isn't in her records," than spend any time paying attention to that data or in discussing the matter with family.

There are times when the records are so wrong as to be dangerous. Mom's short list of allergies was incorrect. There are only two items; how could they get it wrong? In fact, she was given one of the two, and you surely know why. *Data absenta.*

Even more disturbingly, there are occasions when the records are deliberately distorted. I was asked at least two dozen times about the circumstances of Mom's fall. I understand that they wanted to rule out abuse on my part, and I answered repeatedly everything I could. The emergency room staff did not want to admit Mom unless I said she had lost consciousness. She had not done so. Over and over, they asked me to say that she had, claiming that she must have. But she had not. She had lost her balance and had fallen, but she fell talking and never stopped. "I fall, I fall, I blooding, I blooding. Hep me! Get me up!" But her eyes had blackened from the fall on her face directly on her glasses. The staff insisted that black eyes are a clear proof that she lost consciousness, a "fact" her own doctor said had long been known to be a mistaken assumption.

The staff insisted I take her home, and I refused. We waited for hours and hours until someone finally read the X-rays and they admitted her. My taking her home might have killed her. They shrugged that off with, "Maybe not." When the surgeon arrived the next morning, he said to us, "I see that she lost consciousness." I said No. "Yes, she did," he insisted; "it's here in the records." Scream.

~ Little Things Mean Way Too Much

The little things I am thinking about are mostly items on nursing home bills. I don't know how pervasive the practice of gouging residents may be, but I do know that it pays to be vigilant and cost conscious and to call the institutional accounting office whenever you think there is a mistake. In our case, nine times out of ten there really was a mistake and never in our favor.

Take a little thing like a bed pad. How much should a resident be charged. At today's discount store prices, I can buy my mother a box of one hundred and twenty for about twenty-three dollars. I pay the same twenty-three dollars for sixty disposable undergarments. How much would I be paying if I still bought them through the nursing home? A minimum of one dollar and as much as two dollars per item. That is an incredible one hundred and twenty dollars to as much as two hundred and forty dollars for something that costs twenty-three! Ask why the exorbitant markup and you may get the same answer that I did: "We charge extra to put them on her." What are we paying roughly five thousand dollars a month for? Surely personal care is included? If you are the financial custodian of a person in a nursing home, make sure you understand what you can bring in and then determine how worthwhile it is to you to let the institution provide the supplies instead. Then make sure that those pads and briefs are really used on your family member, not distributed to anyone who just happens to need either or both– and especially watch those room mates.

Take a smaller thing: a pill. Most nursing home residents are on a variety of medications, and it is reasonable to take safety precautions with those meds. I accept that it is necessary to have individually wrapped tablets and capsules, although I notice that not everything really is security-wrapped. The nursing home itself provides liquid medications that anyone can contaminate or use for others, and it also provides some tablets that have no safety wrapping. We had to discard six hundred dollars' worth of medications that had been prescribed for Mom only a few days prior to her entering the nursing home, but we had not been told that she could not make use of a single one of them. It also pays to check under beds and in wastebaskets to make sure that none of the medications has landed outside the resident. But the important point is that you have every right to purchase prescriptions and over the counter items from outside the institutional system, as long as the products meet the requirements. Switching from the in-house pharmacy to a chain store pharmacy reduced Mom's monthly meds bill from a minimum of four hundred dollars per month to under one hundred and twenty-five. One specific medication dropped from ninety eight dollars per month to eleven dollars. I called the in-house pharmacy to challenge their billing, and they assured me that the chain store was violating the law. I checked prices online, and I discovered that there is a huge range of prices for that prescription but that the low end eleven dollars was common while the ninety eight dollar price tag was extreme and unusual. I'd call the system criminal.

Take a bigger thing: medical equipment such as an oxygen tank or a nebulizer. We were billed for three months of use of a nebulizer that Mom had used for less than a week. Sometimes, because of the record-keeping problems, it will be hard to prove what you know to be true. Don't give up the fight. We got a refund on the nebulizer– which, by the way, they acknowledged after the fact that she hadn't needed in the first place.

Take things that you bring in for your resident. Or, rather, don't take them. Items of clothing were frequently gone in less than a week. It took a while but finally my sister, learning a lesson from the experts, began billing the nursing home for replacing "lost" apparel. The chest of drawers in my mother's room fills up regularly with articles clearly labeled with other residents' names. They neither are Mom's nor are they usable. They may or may not belong to now-deceased residents; but, whatever the source, she is not in need of other women's bras or underpants. Furthermore, she cannot be made to fit into size 32s; it just isn't possible, although some aides do try. I have found her on many occasions with a bra resting on her shoulders because it was too small to fit normally.

Some of the problems originate in the laundry room. Clothes may go there clearly labeled in permanent marker, but clarity only matters if the personnel can read. Mom gets lots of clothes that have names starting with her same initial. Room numbers on the clothing seem to mean nothing.

These are not necessary problems. They occur partly out of carelessness and partly out of disinterest but too often out of common institutional greed and exploitation. Medicare, always asking us consumers to be vigilant, seems in fact to discourage the practice. I have called to ask for itemized statements so that I know if they are being billed for items of care actually received. The person I spoke with assured me that they checked such things out and that there was no need for me to call. She is wrong. I know that Medicare has been billed for services that we had refused. How does Medicare think it knows?

Once in a while they do check, and they did so for my "blood" aunt. They refused to pay for all radiation treatments administered after my aunt's death. The bill came to me. I called the hospital billing office and explained that no one was going to pay for those fourteen extra treatments not administered. "But she was signed up for them," the billing person said. I explained again that she had not lived to receive them. Billing Lady said she would have to look into it. I suggested that she simply look at my aunt's records and see that her date of death was roughly a week after the series of treatments had begun. The woman thought it would be simpler if we just went ahead and paid the bill. I don't think so.

~ It Doesn't Take a Crystal Ball

Back in that first week that Mom came home with me, her doctor had strongly suggested that she needed to lose some weight. She had a history of high blood pressure and was about thirty pounds over what he thought good for her. I could stand to lose about fifteen, so we embarked on our own program together. The first thing to go was the degree of salt she had always used in cooking. It now became a very small amount, and I used more pepper, for example, in her scrambled eggs and no salt at all. We both love bread and potatoes– carbs are so satisfying– but we cut down on them, too. Over the next three months we both lost ten pounds, a slow steady rate. The nurse who came to the house to check her blood pressure was pleased to report that it was at a very comfortable level.

By the end of a few more months, Mom had lost a total of twenty pounds and I had lost fifteen. We liked the more comfortable fit of our clothes, but best of all was her blood pressure result. Her doctor was pleased; we both thought her new weight was good news in every way. Mom and I kept the pounds off the whole three years.

When she entered the nursing facility, I was asked about her diet; and I asked them to keep her on the light-salt program and mentioned her weight level. The goal was to maintain that weight, not regain it. They told me that at her age, weight was not significant. Family agreed. They said, "Let her enjoy her food; what else does she have to give her pleasure?" In less than three months Mom was up eleven pounds, and her blood pressure had crept up too.

I don't think it takes a crystal ball to see the negative possibilities of their thinking or lack of thinking. Their stated attitude was, If she strokes out, she strokes out. My attitude was, If she "strokes" but not "out" and loses what capabilities she still has, we have compounded the misery and tragedy. It is not pleasurable to have high blood pressure and be subject to massive hemorrhaging, as she is. It is not pleasant at all to feel perpetually uncomfortable. It is scary to have strokes, large or small. The risks were high.

Despite the fact that two of her medications stipulated no alcohol, a few people thought Mom should not be deprived of the "fun" of having an occasional glass of wine. Wine might be "fun" if it didn't have serious consequences for her; but after one glass of wine when out with others, she awoke the next morning with blood coagulated in both eyes. She never wanted wine again, and she shouldn't have had it then. It was, however, very interesting that she remembered what had happened and refused wine thereafter. Don't ask me what the fun was; I don't know.

Back at the nursing home no one cared about the weight gain; but the minute she lost some of that excess poundage, they were on the phone to me to let me know that weight loss was unacceptable. They wanted to increase her caloric intake, and we fought. I lost. Her loss of weight made their required reports to various agencies look bad. It appeared as if they were depriving her of food.

Well, that is what it's all about, isn't it? We can ignore the patient's real needs as long as the results do not tarnish the image of the care she is receiving. Nurses or aides can leave her soiled for hours at a time as long as they are able to report using a reasonable number of undergarments. They can fail to take her to a meal, if she isn't losing weight. They can wake her at a ridiculously early hour when she needs to sleep. They can put eight bedpads under her instead of one or two, if they charge family by the number, or one pad instead of eight if family isn't being charged. They also can lie.

Sometimes I will get a call from the nursing staff to request permission to increase the dosage of tranquilizer Mom takes or to authorize a strong sedative. Why? "She's feisty today and not cooperating with us." My answer is always No. I will not give them permission to take away her ability to express her indignation at how they are caring for her, and that is the issue. When she feels respected and well-tended, she is affectionate and cooperative with them; but when she feels mistreated and put upon, she will find a way to make her reactions known. I will not let them drug her out of self-expression, especially not simply for their convenience. "Take better care of her," I say, "and that will solve the problem."

It doesn't take a crystal ball to see all too fearfully that the current direction of health care for the elderly– really for all of us– will only continue to go against human interests and remain all about corporate interests. And yet a crystal ball could be really helpful to let these institutions and their managers and staff see the eventual outcome: ever more depersonalization and inhumanity and increasing detachment from true service. For all the current love affair with accountability, we don't have it at all. Yes, of course there are exceptions, thank goodness, but not enough of them.

The ball could be just as helpful for individuals who fail to see the consequences of even small things like a glass of wine or an extra piece of pie. If they can't see the potential harm in what they propose, at least they could accept major visual aids. "Look closely. Here is what your action is likely to produce. Think before you act, and don't overvalue spontaneity when dealing with another person's life." I don't see it happening, but it would be wonderful to be wrong.

I See You ~ ~

I see you there
from here behind my eyes.
You think I do not know or hear,

as I lie here,
or understand your truths, your lies.

I call that one my mother;
I know she's not.
The words come out the way they want,
not how I want;
inside my head they're caught.

You tell her what you want to say,
like, "She has not been good."
It's you who treat me like a block,
a block of wood,
and not the way you should.

Oh, let me out of here, I say;
let me go where I want to be.
My love lies in a far-off field
beneath a stone.
Too long he's been alone;
too long I've been alone.
He waits for me
so patiently,
and I would be with him.

~ The Forest Primeval (a continuation of "Mother Tongue")

All that charted territory we call the brain continues to hold its own deep mysteries. Scientists probe the structures and map centers and functions within it, but how much that is current knowledge is accurate? How much do they understand? Among the kinds of television shows I do try to watch, documentaries about the brain come high on the list. I look for anything that will help me understand the contradictions and problems my mother posed and still continues to pose.

I know they can do intricate surgery to isolate and remove certain tumors while doing by current standards the least possible damage. I am confident that those standards will change dramatically in our favor, that surgeons and researchers will develop ever more sophisticated techniques to conquer devastating brain damage. Almost all of my questions revolve around a single point: is what you know true? Surely my mother is not the only exception to your rules, so how can I believe that your prognosis and advice are based on accurate assumptions and

94

knowledge? How can I trust you?

I think of one of my nieces who did undergo surgery for a brain tumor. She stayed awake during the process in order to be able to help the team of doctors and nurses know their own progress. She came through the ordeal in what was a near-miraculous success. How can I not trust that medicine does have some answers right? The fact is, every situation is uniquely its own. The individual makes all the difference– the individual patient and each individual member of the medical team.

I think of the social worker in the first days of our in-house stroke journey (see "Mother, Humphrey, Dog") and her insistence that Mom was incapable of rational thought or intelligent responses. That person represents the worst side of medical guidance. With no knowledge of the patient or the caregiver, she proceeded to dictate ridiculous rules and arbitrary, mechanical responses to a variety of situations. One must at times yield to the professionals, but then one must also stand one's ground.

I think of my mother, hearing one family member tell another how much she was doing for Mom; and I smiled as she winked at me, shook her head, rolled her eyes, and whispered, "She liar." I think of the little plans she conceived to get her way; the reasons she presented, however manipulative and transparent, to get me to change my mind about going or not going out on a particular day; the techniques she tried out to get my visitors to leave. Whether or not she was successful, she was still thinking. She was more childlike in her methods, but she still knew what she wanted. Unfortunately, what she wanted was total control, and that goal was not attainable.

Today I laugh a little at her greeting me in the nursing home hall, grabbing my arm, and pulling me down so that she can whisper, "We get out of here now. We go get a little food. I go home with you." Sad as it is to dash her hopes, there is no way I can say Yes; but don't tell me her brain isn't working.

Watch her eyes dart from domino to domino as she develops a sound strategy to win. She can remember long enough what numbers I do not have on my tiles, and she is a joyously chortling winner most of the time. Yes, she can think ahead and plan.

Tell me that that the scan of her brain shows massive damage, and I believe you; but tell me that she is therefore completely mentally incompetent, and it's you I will challenge. Stop believing everything you read and every statistic that tumbles into your path. Look at the real person and figure out, at the very least, what is compensating for what.

Believe if you want that she does not know what she is saying, that there is nothing left for her to think with; but something is working. If all else appears destroyed, somewhere she retains the memory of how to manipulate. Her success rate isn't what it was, but tell me where that function resides in the brain– it clearly isn't in the massively damaged area. Don't dismiss her as a fluke; look to her as an example of what might still survive.

Somebod' Listen ~ ~

I mad at him.
I thought he good.
I tell him take me home,
but he say here is it.
I scheme at mother,
who make me stay.
Did I say he?
*Why **she** not listen me?*

Why she keep me in this place
where evbody so old?
They cannot talk or walk;
like little nakkins they all fold,
like new wrap paper rolled.
But I still young
at ninety-five.
I still alive.
To me she cold.
To me she dead.

Go home.
That all that on my mind.
Don't look for me
in prison chair,
no me here will you find.

She do not listen, she not care;
so I will keep on scream to God,
"O, bring me home."
Why no one hear?

~ Hospice

I was working at school when I received a call from Mom's doctor's assistant, the one who made most of the nursing home visits and checked on her fairly regularly. It was not too long after she had fallen trying to get out of her wheelchair and had sustained a painful fracture. Her recovery required her to stay in bed for several weeks, having all her meals there, and moving as little as possible other than slightly shifting positions to avoid bed sores (which she did not avoid at all). Her spirits were extremely low, hardly surprising, and she lost appetite and weight. She tried to will herself to death, but it just did not work.

Barry's call was to ask me if I would be surprised if he said she was dying. The fact is that I would not have been surprised to hear that at any time during the months, now years, since her stroke. I told him that I would not but also that I would not be surprised if she rallied and regained her former status. Her resilience remained remarkable.

Barry explained that her degree of decline and her significant loss of weight and appetite made her a plausible candidate for hospice care. My not being surprised at the thought of her dying just added to the probability that she could be enrolled. I was okay with that, although I think that family attitude should be considered of worth but not always definitive. At any rate, she did enroll in hospice; and finally I came to have some respect for medical care.

She did not receive daily visits, but she did have a few visits each week. I received weekly communications on her state of being– a first. Only the necessary medications were administered. Her personal care really did become what its name implied: personal. She was bathed with greater gentleness; her hair care suited her better– gently massaged shampoos and styling the way she liked. She was given help when she needed it and allowed to be independent where she could safely be so. She was treated wholeheartedly like a valuable human being, and so we know the outcome.

She started eating; she gained back some weight. She recovered from her injuries enough to be able to get into her chair again. She resumed having a slight interest in other residents, though not more than she had previously shown. She graduated from hospice, not to a higher world. A few months later, you would not have guessed she had been through any ordeal.

She has hospice care to thank for her life or blame it for keeping her here. Either way, the hospice workers are people to appreciate and welcome, and the hospice program is one to be emulated in regular medical care.

~ Chocolate Is Just Dessert

If anyone is handing out treats, make mine chocolate, please. Many things can sweeten the day, but good chocolate can be available at any time and with or without company. You don't need a partner. I do like treats and I regularly provide them, but just desserts are another thing entirely. I'd like to abolish the whole idea.

Ever since I entered the caregiver role, there have been plenty of kind, well-meaning people– friends and strangers alike– who want to assure me that I deserve and will have a just reward. They like to assure me of a shining spot in their heaven. We say such things to people we like, admire, respect, or agree with. Those we dislike, fail to admire, cannot respect, or disagree with we tend to assume deserve nothing good; in fact, we tend to consign them to hell. I cringe when anyone tells me what I deserve, and I would erase that word and send it to oblivion in the larger package of just desserts. I don't believe that what I have done leads automatically to anything at all, other than the lessons I draw from my experiences. What we learn is either our reward or punishment; it is what ultimately matters.

In the same way, those who assured me that Mom did not deserve to be cared for at home are too caught up in reward and punishment and fail to see that there are things all people of every degree of good or evil are entitled to have. Whether they get those things or not is another matter, but no one is rejectable unless all of us are. No one is undeserving of care, and therefore deserving is a nonissue.

I have been challenged on this belief. People will remind me of the many villains of the world. What about them? they ask. Well, what about them? Do we know what led them to their behavior? Did they start out villainous? Who warped them and why? Was it a failure of caring on someone else's part? Was it neglect and lack of love, lack of respect? Do we have to reject them because they could not give what they had never received? What about the power monsters? What leads anyone to the belief that position and money confer rights over the lives and deaths of others? The reality through history has been that some have inexcusable power, while others have to live in excruciating powerlessness over even their daily acts and thoughts. Does the word "deserve" really apply?

So many of us have been indoctrinated with the idea that good deeds get rewarded and bad deeds get punished. Well, sometimes that's the case; more often it isn't. The saying, no good deed goes unpunished, reflects our more realistic observations. All of this is moot. If I were handing out just desserts, I'd have to give the giant's share to those who loved and provided all along, not to those of us who came late to the bedside. Yet there is room for all of us and ways that all of us can lay claim to at least a bonbon, if not a whole box of candy. Reward us all for living in this world of suffering and cruelty, and especially acknowledge that the original goodies were never distributed equally. Life does not appear to operate on this plan of just desserts; it gives some a seven-course meal and others a spoon of watered soup.

I don't pretend that I know what, if anything, comes next. I have my hopes and fears, but I don't have an assured knowing. I do know that the image of stars in one's crown, however beautiful, holds little reality for me. Deserve? Such a simple concept. Very human but way too simple. We are such a mix of things chemical and parts biological and factors psychological and yearnings spiritual and beliefs self-preservational and issues comical– maybe, for all I know, even karmical– how do we separate and understand them at all?

What I have learned repeatedly in my life, what has become a central theme, is also simple: we do what our specific life calls upon us to do. Or we refuse. I believe that life is about experience, that we are part of a tremendous dynamic relationship in which That Which Knows learns. Every shade of every possibility will be explored in time, and every drop of knowledge and experience expands God and humanity. Whether it is science or art or philosophy or the psychology of behavior or television cartoons, all is grist for the life force to convert potential to real. Good and evil hold equal weight on a cosmic level, however untrue personally. No life is excluded from the plan.

"Deserve" is irrelevant. "Just dessert" is a really good chocolate bar.

~ The Difference a "Deem" Makes

One of the ironic impacts of living with language loss is that the caregiver is apt to acquire a whole new subvocabulary. "Pencil" as a noun that means anything and everything is one example. Every time I hear someone use that word, I experience a very brief sense of displacement. "What," I am likely to think, "does he really mean?" The flash passes, and I know he means *pencil*. Imagine that!

On my mother's good language days, which tend to come in brief batches and then dissolve, I am usually able to figure out what possible rhyming word or near-miss word she really does mean. On a recent trip to the nursing home, I found her fast asleep and not easy to arouse. Clearly startled and at first unwilling to open her eyes, she waved her arms all around as if to regain her balance and at last blinked herself awake. I would not have been surprised to hear her launch into sleepy absolutely incoherent sounds, but no. As I slowly came into focus, she got more and more excited to see me. She reached out to pull me into a hug. No *pencil, pencil, pencil* came tumbling out of her mouth. Instead, she joyously called out, "I just this min deeming about you! I deem about us and here you."

It is the kind of event that gives a glow to the day and smiles to my eyes. Think of how it would have been to hear, "I pencil you, I just this pencil been pencil you." There would have been no shine in my eyes, nor in hers either.

It is ever more remarkable to me each time it happens. It seems a miracle of brain cells, an absolute case of some very generous sandman having sprinkled word dust over her and enabled her to speak in loving ways. On my previous visit she had not spoken to me at all except to vent her fury that I was once again not taking her home with me. I do thank God and sandmen for allowing her mind to forget each time and to be a surprise to me at every visit.

Sometimes on a day when she has dreamed about us, she thinks it is magic that I really do appear. "How you know?" she will ask. "How you know to find me here now? I so afaid you nev fine me again." Is it a terrible thing to encourage her belief that I somehow sense when she is calling to me? I hope not. In the first place, it often is true; but even when I am blind to her needs and deaf to her calls, I finally see our hard-won relationship as a very strong one. Tomorrow she may not know me or care; but on the days that she does both know and care, she is overflowing with happiness and the real kisses and the deep hugs I went so long without.

I deem each wondrous time a gift of love.

~ Almost the Last Word

~ I Say

You valiant are,
sturdy, strong,
with traits I do admire;
but never will I be like you,
never shall aspire
to all that you have come to be–
I lack your Aries home-hearth fire.

I have a sturdiness of my own,
strength of a different kind.
I'd rather climb my goat-like path
on mountains capped with ice
than set my dreams in kitchens
and measure life by "nice".
Yet nice it is, amazing too,
that we have come this far –
that we can love each other,
no matter who we are.

She Says ~ ~

I still not close as I can get
to home which where I want to be.
My days too long,
my life too short;
my mother old as me.
It still confuzzing
when I talk,
confuzzing what I hear.
I think she say she love me now.
I think to her I dear.
These not words I am used to see
when this one speak to me.
So guess we love together now.
It miracle to me.

~ Hugs and Kisses, Words of Love

Perhaps I should have placed this essay at the beginning of this book, but I like it here at the end. I am trying to remember the first time that I heard the words *I love you* from my mother. I think I was in my thirties, and I know I assumed because she wasn't looking directly at me that she thought I was my sister. Our family was more than a little paradoxical about emotions. Everybody hugged and kissed us all and kissed each other warmly without regard to gender. The men were not embarrassed to kiss their brothers or fathers or everybody's wives, but expressing affection in words was simply not done. Saying loving things to children especially was bad for their humility quotient. You wouldn't want a child to think too much of himself. Even the physical hugs and other expressions of love were often followed by joking insults, and not all of us can keep from internalizing the insults and feeling that they override the affection. I grew up feeling somewhat loved some of the time, not a great base of security but better than no love at all.

Mostly it was the genuine warmth and kindness of my maternal grandparents and one of my uncles and one of my aunts, along with the depth of love I felt from my father, that provided what comfort I had. My mother was never such a source– little affection, no endearing terms except to my sister; but no one at all was verbal on the topic.

I had very mixed reactions to all this. On one hand, the hugs and kisses were like a pot about to boil; on the other hand, the lack of words cooled everything well below the bubbling point. The elderly great aunts and uncles made lack of affection okay; being hugged was bad enough, but being kissed was painful. Between sharp whiskers and foul breath, their demonstrativeness frequently sent me on lengthy trips to the second floor of the house long before they were ready to leave– I knew they couldn't climb steps. Someone would call me down to kiss Aunt Sophie goodbye or get a fierce whisker burn from Uncle Will, and I would pretend to be asleep. Occasionally it worked, not often. Hiding in the bathroom did not work either. One or another of my parents would threaten to unlock the door and bring the troops in.

This is not to say that I didn't want hugs and kisses, just not from some of them. I became slightly elder-hostile, except for the few I have already mentioned. Yet to this day it seems odd to me that no one ever *told* us that they loved us. We took it for granted when we felt a little bit secure and felt unentitled to the words when we felt lost or lonely. Perhaps I am speaking only for myself; possibly my siblings heard those words regularly or possibly they had very different reactions. Maybe only the black sheep was excluded from endearments. However, since for me warmth was very slow to evolve, I turned elsewhere. Mostly I turned to books and to school.

Books– what rescuers they were! How grateful I was that there were people who could put strong feelings into words and share them with me! For some of us, words are the most meaningful conveyers of reality. Hugs and kisses, yes, they are so important; but they can become at least as formulaic as some people find language. How very unpleasant it is to be hugged by someone who is about to tell you something that hurts. How difficult it is to accept kisses from someone who has just been explaining your faults.

I have heard that too rare phrase *I love you* many times now from my mother, more in the seven years since her stroke than in the fifty-seven years prior to it. They soften my heart toward her and make her major aggravations more tolerable but also more sad. I don't know why it took so long or why it was so hard. One day when she was feeling particularly expansive, she threw her arms out wide and said to me, "I love evbody. I love evbody. Even you." And despite that pathetic qualifier at the end, I welcomed her words and my eyes could not keep from filling just a little. I could honestly say I loved her too. That day made lots of others endurable. It salvaged something I had thought permanently absent and it began to ease a lifelong need.

My own children may or may not give much thought to how much I tell them I love them, but it matters to me to tell them as often as they will let me. Love unexpressed creates eternal longing, needless trauma, human misery. For some, loving action is the cure and will always be enough; but many of us need the words as well. What better deed can we do for the world than to sing to each other while we can hear?

Future Projects by White Canoe Productions

Jody Lewis

A Greater Disgrace   light mystery

A Herring Sampler   short stories

Jody Lewis and Laura Ziggle

The Tree in the Window   magical realism

ORDER FORM for *Sing To Me While I Can Hear*

Price list for individual or bulk orders

Number of copies	Price per copy
1- 9	$15.00
10 - 25	$12.95
26 - 50	$10.00
51 +	please inquire

Copies .....   Subtotal: ....
MO residents add 7% tax   ....
Shipping/handling - UPS   ..$5.00...

Amount enclosed   ....

Send payment (US) and order form to

    White Canoe Productions
    472 Sunstone Drive
    St. Louis, Missouri 63011-3412

Name...
Street...
City........................... State...... Zip..........

THIS PAGE MAY BE REPRODUCED.

ORDER FORM for *Sing To Me While I Can Hear*

Price list for individual or bulk orders

Number of copies	Price per copy
1- 9	$15.00
10 - 25	$12.95
26 - 50	$10.00
51 +	please inquire

Copies .....   Subtotal: ....
MO residents add 7% tax   ....
Shipping/handling - UPS   ..$5.00...

Amount enclosed   ....

Send payment (US) and order form to

White Canoe Productions
472 Sunstone Drive
St. Louis, Missouri 63011-3412

Name...
Street..
City.. State...... Zip..........

THIS PAGE MAY BE REPRODUCED.